What people are s
LIVING WITH A DEAF DOG

"...every so often a book comes along that hits on such a timely subject that is deserves some extra attention. Filled with facts and advice from deaf-dog owners and canine professionals from around the world, *Living With A Deaf Dog* helps disprove myths and gives hope and encouragement to people who own these special animals."
—*Donna L. Marcel, Editor/DogWorld Magazine*

"How profoundly touched I was by *Living With A Deaf Dog*. What a splendid, readable and thoroughly professional book."
—*Susan Moldow, Vice President & Publisher/Scribner*

Living With A Deaf Dog includes two informative chapters (How To Communicate With Your Deaf Dog and Deaf Dog Traits, Training and Safety Tips) which will help guardians of deaf dogs train, communicate with and help keep their hearing impaired canines safe.
—*N. Glenn Perrett, Writer/PETS Magazine*

"When I ordered the book, I thought that maybe there wouldn't be any information that was new to me because I have owned deaf dogs for almost five years....but was I wrong! My copy is already dog-eared!"
—*Holly Newstead/Founder and Director of*
  Deaf Dog Education Action Fund/Deaf Dog Owner

"Susan Cope Becker 's new book is a wonderful read! I get many calls from around the country on deaf Danes and NOW I have a book to steer them to instead of just my experiences."
—*Sandy Suarez/Great Dane Rescue, Inc/Deaf Dog Owner*

LIVING WITH A DEAF DOG

A book of advice, facts
and experiences
about canine deafness

SUSAN COPE BECKER

Illustrations by Andy Caylor

Published by
Susan Cope Becker

Published by
Susan Cope Becker
2555 Newtown Road
Cincinnati, Ohio 45244

First Edition/1997
Second Printing/March, 1998
Third Printing/January, 2000

Manufactured in the United States

Library of Congress Catalog Card Number: 97-094306

Susan Cope Becker
Living With A Deaf Dog

ISBN : 0-9660058-0-5

This book is dedicated to my mom,
who taught me how to love and be kind to animals;

to all of the people who have
opened their hearts and minds
to the lovable and noble deaf dog;

and to Spanky–
my loyal and constant companion.

*Nothing is impossible
to a willing heart.*

John Heywood
1546

AN IMPORTANT NOTE
FROM THE AUTHOR

This book has not been written to popularize owning a deaf dog. I am not promoting a fad. Deaf dogs are not a novelty. Owning any dog–hearing or deaf, mixed breed or pedigreed–is a serious commitment that requires compassion, patience, kindness, understanding and devotion. Owning a deaf dog requires a little more of all of these. And if you have never owned and trained a dog, I do not recommend your first dog be a deaf one.

ACKNOWLEDGMENTS

This book reflects the experience of hundreds of people who live with deaf dogs. They are the folks I met on the Internet when I desperately went in search of advice on how to train and communicate with Spanky. They are the folks with whom I shared my own tips and experience. They have become friends without faces, but friends with lots of heart and sound information. And they have never let me forget that I made a commitment to do this book, and have encouraged me to keep on even when I slowed to a complete halt. From these wonderful, compassionate folks, I have gathered extensive files of e-mail communications and bulletin board postings that record hundreds of training tips, hand signs, and experiences about life with a deaf dog.

I will forever be grateful to the first people I talked with about deafness in dogs, many of whom shared articles and correspondence regarding deaf dogs and canine deafness when I began my research for writing this book. All of them shared their enthusiasm, tips and encouragement when I set about training Spanky: Julie Nelson, Lynn Sickenger, Dr. Michael Sims of the University of Tennessee Department of Small Animal Sciences Veterinary Teaching Hospital, Dr. Michael Moore of Washington State Veterinary College, Michele Dunefsky, Caroline Crosby of the Santa Fe School for Deaf Dalmatians in New Mexico, and Connie Bombaci. Lyndsay Patten deserves recognition and a large thanks from all of us deaf dog owners for setting up the Deaf Dog Web Page and giving of his time and skills to create the Deaf Dog Mailing List where hundreds of us have come together to discuss everything from how to say *no*, to deaf dog rescues, to separation anxiety, to the injustices the deaf dog faces in today's world. I must thank the hundreds of people who took the time to fill out questionnaires that so much of my research is based upon.

My gratitude to M.L. Tanner who referred me to Amber Saunders of Four Paws training school in Lenoir City, Tennessee who had never trained a deaf dog, but who didn't say no to trying. Not only did she try, she succeeded and Spanky rewarded her by graduating number two in the class.

Heartfelt thanks to Lyn Diable who is the owner of Kushti Dalmatian Club and

Animal Sanctuary in West Sussex, England. I feel like we're old friends. She shared stacks of her newsletters, distributed my questionnaire, gave my information to Britain's *Dog World* magazine for publication, and shared so much of her knowledge and experiences with me.

Dr. George Strain of Louisiana State University has spent years researching deafness and never hesitated to share his information and knowledge. Without him, this book would not have been complete.

Appreciation goes to all of my family members and friends (old and new) who accept Spanky just as she is, and who took the time to learn Spanky's sign language so they, too, can communicate with her. Thanks to my son David who provided Spanky with patience, love and her first canine playmate, Maddie. Love and gratitude goes to my husband Ethan for loving Spanky from the beginning, listening when I talked incessantly about canine deafness, and for always encouraging me to get this book finished. He supported my efforts and tolerated my absences as I sat hours in front of the computer, with my head in the manuscript, or on the phone with deaf dog owners, dog lovers and experts.

A special thanks to my mom, Sue Anderson (Spanky's granny), Anne Daniels and Mary Gilbert who dog-sit when Ethan and I travel; an extra thank you to Mary for her valuable assistance on getting this book finished; and appreciation to Susan Collins, mom, Anne, and Mary for proofing the book and offering sound editorial advice. Thanks to Andy Caylor for his incredible illustrations that will help so many deaf dogs and their owners communicate. My gratitude also goes to Chris Reed who was a great training partner in Spanky's earliest days and who encouraged me when I considered writing this book.

Last but certainly not least, I must thank Spanky, for if not for her, I would have remained totally unaware of the deaf canine population and their very special owners. I would not know the joy that all God's creatures know whether they are hearing or deaf. She has brought me a much more open heart and mind.

Susan Cope Becker
September, 1997

TABLE OF
CONTENTS

FOREWORD

I am not an expert dog trainer. I am not an animal behaviorist. I am a writer by profession, however, and the owner of a deaf dog. And with those two qualifications, I have undertaken the task of writing this book.

This book has been written because I don't want another deaf dog owner to feel the hopelessness and fear of loss that I experienced when I discovered my brand new puppy was deaf. Instead, I want anyone who goes searching for information on deaf dogs to find it...reliable information on canine deafness, training tips, hand signs, and shared stories from other deaf dog owners with whom they can relate.

Next, I want to create an option that veterinarians and breeders can offer deaf dog owners instead of euthanasia. I also hope to provide dog trainers a book to refer to when they accept a deaf dog into an obedience class. It was important to me to write a book that would allow deaf dog owners everywhere to share their abundance of encouragement and hope with the new deaf dog owner. And finally, I want to increase awareness about dogs who are deaf and the injustices they face because of their special challenge.

To those of you who are just learning about or getting to know a deaf dog, keep these things in mind. Do not pity deaf dogs. They are not in pain. They are not brain damaged. They are not unhappy. Deaf dogs are noble, intelligent and lovable animals.

To those of you who are just beginning the process of training your deaf dogs, I applaud you and am certain your efforts will be greatly rewarded. Good luck.

Susan Cope Becker
September, 1997

INTRODUCTION

When I began doing electrodiagnostic evaluation of audiologic function in animals in 1983, I became keenly aware of the one element that is missing in animals that makes auditory evaluation so much easier in most humans beings, namely verbal communication.

One of the most popular procedures at that time was the auditory brainstem response (ABR) or the brainstem auditory evoked response (BAER, pronounced "bear"). This procedure consisted of using computers to record time-averaged electrical activity from the brain in response to repetitive sound stimulation.

Such procedures are necessary because like animals, not all human beings are able to communicate effectively. This is especially true for human infants, many of whom are evaluated for auditory function within the first postnatal week. At the clinic, we get requests on a regular basis from conscientious breeders as they become aware of the value of BAER testing.

On the basis of BAER testing, some breeders elect to euthanize bilaterally deaf puppies and require the neutering of unilaterally deaf pups. Unfortunately, many of our clients were discovering deafness several weeks or even months after obtaining affected pups. What may have been passed off as immaturity was later realized to be a serious handicap.

In the Department of Small Animal Clinical Sciences in the Veterinary Teaching Hospital at the University of Tennessee, we assumed the responsibility for providing an accurate diagnosis of auditory dysfunction and in many cases provided encouragement and practical advice about owning a deaf dog. At the top of the list of information we warned that deaf dogs can startle easily which can cause aggressive episodes; and explained to their owners that they must take extra measures to protect their dogs from dangers ordinarily accompanied by warning sounds, such as traffic.

Perhaps the greatest challenge facing owners of deaf dogs is how to train their pets to successfully behave and interact with people and other animals without the advantage of verbal commands. Unfortunately, very few resources are available to owners who elect to keep their deaf pets. For years, I have personally encouraged clients to record their observations of successful training techniques so that I could pass them along to others. Some said they would but never did. They were most likely overwhelmed by the level of dedication that was required.

Susan Cope Becker did follow through. In *Living With A Deaf Dog*, Susan is providing what has been needed for a long time–both encouragement and how-to's. She has combined her own personal experiences with those of others in recognition of the diversity that has been used by people from all over the world to train deaf dogs. Without the advantage of readily accessible models, these people have created their own success stories.

I personally believe that these efforts are just the first in a succession of writings aimed at improving the quality of life for handicapped animals and their owners.

Michael Sims, Ph.D.
Physiologist
Department of Small Animal Sciences
Veterinary Teaching Hospital
University of Tennessee

Learning to love and accept that which is different is one of life's great lessons, and for me, Spanky is one of life's great teachers.

CHAPTER ONE
Living with Spanky

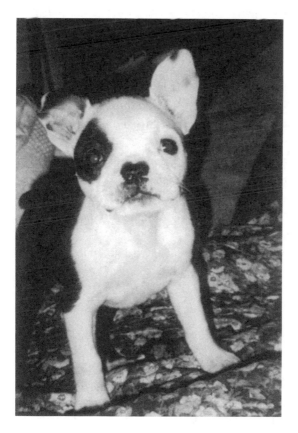

In February of 1995, I bought a beautiful Boston Terrier puppy and named her Spanky. I brought her home on a Thursday evening, and spent most of the time holding her and watching her sleep in my arms or on my lap. When I turned in for the night, I laid her gently beside me in bed where she sleeps to this day.

Being self-employed, I decided to take the next day off and spend it with the new member of the family. I got up early with Spanky and took her outside for her morning bathroom time, fed her and then began my morning routine of coffee and newspaper. When I left the living room to go get another cup of coffee, she was on the sofa and began to cry loudly. I called to her from the kitchen, but the crying persisted. I grabbed my video camera and headed back to the living room talking "puppy talk" to her expecting her to turn and look at me with delight...all of which I would capture on the camcorder.

Instead, she continued crying, facing away from the hallway where I stood. I walked to the center of the room (still taping) and called to her again. Nothing. It wasn't until I put down the camera and went to her and touched her that she turned quickly, and upon seeing me quit crying, began licking my hands and climbing up on my lap. I thought this unusual, but decided she hadn't heard me over her own noise.

A while later, we were playing and Spanky clamped her teeth onto my hand. I felt her needle-sharp teeth penetrating my flesh. Unlike all the other puppies I have had, she did not let go when I cried out and tried to pull away from her. In intense pain and unable to make her let go, I gently struck her head and she finally let go.

Let me stop here and let you know that I have had Boston Terriers since I was eight years old. As an adult, I have had three Bostons, two of which gave me three litters of puppies. I rarely hit a dog as a form of discipline, and I have never had one bite me until I was bleeding.

Needless to say, I was confused by her behavior. I then recalled seeing her bite her litter mate's ear until it began to bleed and all the while the male pup she was biting was emitting an ear-piercing scream. My only rationale was as the biggest puppy in the litter, she had an aggressive nature. But I decided not to worry. I could train her to be gentle.

Throughout the morning I saw many behaviors exhibited that indicated a dog who couldn't or wouldn't listen to me. Could she be deaf? What an incredibly hopeless thought! I had never heard of a deaf dog and couldn't imagine how a deaf dog could be trained or live a normal life. I decided to "test" her.

When Spanky went to sleep, I whistled over her head and she woke up. I squeaked a toy behind her and she turned around. I clapped my hands over her head as she napped and she woke up. I decided I was wrong. She could hear me and was just a stubborn, little character.

Saturday came and went and on Sunday, I began doubting my tests. I went out and bought a dog whistle which I blew until my face was blue. No reaction from Spanky. I then remembered the video I had shot of her crying so loudly on Friday morning. I cued it up, pressed play and turned up the volume. She never even look toward the television. Then I tried the ultimate test.

I held her with her back to the vacuum cleaner and turned it on. She didn't jump or shy away from the noise. Then I turned her around to face it and she ran and jumped up on it to examine this new object. She showed absolutely no fear of a machine that causes most hearing animals to head for the hills.

I was finally convinced that she was deaf, and realized that my earlier tests had fooled me because she was feeling the air movement from my hands clapping together, or the air from the squeaky toy or my whistles. Because it was late, I couldn't call a veterinarian, so I called a friend who is a veterinary student at the University of Tennessee. She pulled out her text books and read aloud to me, "...aggressive litter mates, often absence of pigment (see Spanky's picture), congenital deafness occurs most often..." She then read the sentence that knocked the wind out of me. The text book recommended that deaf dogs be euthanized warning of aggression and difficulty in training them. When I hung up the phone, I held Spanky close to me and wept. I decided I would find a way to deal with this and I would not, under any circumstances, put Spanky to sleep.

I called the breeders whom I have known for years. They were very sorry and said I could return Spanky for a refund or another puppy, but that simply was not an option. I loved her, deaf or not. Spanky's great-great grandparents had been Soccer and Roxanne, my dame and sire of long ago, and her similarity to Roxi created yet another level of attachment for me.

Never in my life had I heard of a deaf Boston Terrier. And as I said before, I really wasn't aware of deafness in dogs at all. But I was soon to find out that deafness in dogs does happen and happens much more often than you would think. And to my disappointment, I was to discover there was little or no information on how to train or communicate with a deaf dog.

Being a writer, I love research. And research I did. But again, I found nothing. Not in the library or the pet catalogs. My veterinarian had never had a deaf dog as a patient and had no training advice, but he did track down a veterinarian at the University of Tennessee who has a sister in Florida with a deaf dog. I called her and she gave me hope. She had successfully trained her Dalmatian with hand signs. Then the breeder called and told me about someone locally who had a deaf Boxer. I called her and she told me the story of her dog and that she also trained her to hand signs.

Because it seemed to me that Spanky heard sounds on occasion (i.e., children on the playground behind our house), our veterinarian recommended I take her to the University of Tennessee School for Veterinary Medicine for the

Brain Auditory Evoked Response test. The BAER test, he explained, is the same test used on humans with hearing problems and deafness. It measures what, if any, level of hearing the person or animal has. The results, however, confirmed that Spanky is totally deaf in both ears.

M.L. Tanner, the technician who administers the BAER test for UT, gave me the name of a trainer in the area that might work with me to train Spanky. Dr. Michael Sims, the physiologist who analyzes the tests, talked at length with me. He gave me copies of two articles he had on deaf dogs which included an address for Santa Fe School for Deaf Dalmatians. But when I asked for written training information, he had nothing to offer.

When I told Dr. Sims that I was thinking about writing a book about owning and training a deaf dog, he encouraged me. He told me such a book was terribly needed and would hopefully save the lives of many deaf dogs since most are senselessly put to sleep, a job with which he was all to familiar.

After that, I wrote the Santa Fe school and ordered their book. There are five wonderful pages on training tips including written descriptions of nine hand signs to use. But I was still thirsty for more so I turned to the Internet. That's where I met many deaf dog owners and received probably the most valuable tip of all: buy a pocketbook version of American Sign Language. With this book in hand, I suddenly felt like I could actually communicate with Spanky. All I had to do was teach her to understand hand signs instead of vocal commands, and that's just what I did with the help of Amber Saunders, the trainer who had been recommended.

While she had never trained a deaf dog, she was willing to learn with me, and she was open to all the information that I had researched and compiled. I gave her copies of the basic signs that I was using: *good girl, stop, no.* She taught me the standard obedience signs used in training dogs: *sit, down, stay, come, heel.* Amber first conducted private sessions with us and was so impressed with Spanky's progress that she recommended I attend a regular class with Spanky to teach her to socialize and obey in the midst of activities with other dogs present. Spanky trained with about eight hearing dogs and was second in the class when she graduated.

Spanky is a well-behaved dog who is loved and accepted. Most people (after being around her for a few hours) are convinced that she isn't completely deaf. She appears to be perfect. Her best friend was my son David's black female Chow, Maddie who was lost to us this past winter. The two of them would run, romp, wrestle, growl, bark, tug, nap, eat and drink together. She now has a stepsister, a German Short Hair Pointer named Joy. She socializes easily with other animals and they all exhibit incredible patience with her, seeming to be aware that she's somehow different from them.

Spanky now knows about 20 signs. And as we sign to her, we talk. Not only is it a natural thing to do, I believe it helps her read facial expressions and body language. While she certainly isn't a guard dog, at two and a half years old, she now "feels" people walk up on the porch, the door open, or cars idle in the driveway sometimes before we hear the doorbell.

She vacations with us on the beach, in the mountains, and travels between Ohio and Tennessee regularly. We walk, go for rides in the car and visit friends at their homes...just like a hearing dog.

Spanky is part of a video that was produced by the University of Tennessee for use in training new veterinary students and owners of deaf dogs about the possibilities that are open to deaf dogs and their owners.

Her limits are few. She lives her life outside on a leash or in a fenced yard. She runs boundary free only on our eight acres in Cincinnati and for short romps on the beach or in the mountains far from harm's way. All in all, Spanky is a lucky dog. And it has been my good fortune to have her come into my life.

She is a constant reminder to me that being "normal" isn't the only acceptable way to be. We all have our handicaps whether you can see them or not. Learning to love and accept that which is different is one of life's greatest lessons, and for me, Spanky is one of life's greatest teachers.

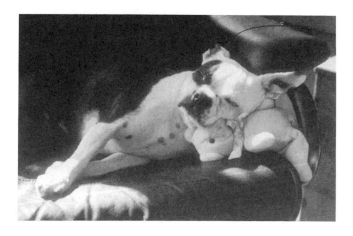

...the myths are that deaf dogs cannot be trained, and they are aggressive, unpredicatable and brain damaged.

CHAPTER TWO

Deafness in Dogs–
Genetics and Temperament

Tens of thousands of deaf dogs are born every year all over the world. This little known fact has little impact until you find yourself loved by and loving an adorable deaf puppy. The advice most often given is to put the dog to sleep. Why? Because the myths are that deaf dogs cannot be trained, they are aggressive, unpredictable and are brain damaged.

Dalmatians have the highest percentage of deafness of any breed. Estimated occurrence of bilateral deafness (deaf in both ears) in Dalmatians ranges from 8% to 16%. The average of the two (12%) is what I have read most recently and use in my calculations in this book.

WHAT CAUSES DEAFNESS IN DOGS?

Congenital deafness is caused by a defective gene. Acquired deafness is caused by a variety of problems. First, a discussion on congenital deafness. Dr. George Strain, Ph.D., Professor of Neuroscience at the School of Veterinary Medicine and Associate Vice Chancellor for Research and Economic Development at Louisiana State University in Baton Rouge has done extensive research on deafness in dogs and cats.

He reported the following in the British Veterinary Journal, Volume 152, pages 17-36 in 1996: "Congenital deafness has been reported for approximately 64 breeds, with the list growing at a regular rate. It can potentially appear in any breed. The deafness has often been long-established in a breed but kept hidden from outsiders to protect reputations. The disorder is usually associated with pigmentation patterns, where increasing amounts of white in the hair coat increase the likelihood of deafness. Two pigmentation genes in particular are often associated with deafness in dogs: the merle gene (seen in the Collie, Shetland Sheepdog, Dappled Dachshund, Harlequin Great Dane, American Foxhound, Old English Sheepdog, Dappled Dunkerhounds among others); and the piebald gene (common in the Bull Terrier, Samoyed, Greyhound, Great Pyrenees, Beagle, Bulldog, Dalmatian, English Setter). The deafness, which usually develops in the first few weeks after birth while the ear canal is still closed, usually results from the degeneration of part of the blood supply to the cochlea (the stria vascularis). The nerve cells of the cochlea subsequently die and permanent deafness results. The cause of the vascular degeneration is not known, but appears to be associated with the absence of pigment producing cells (melanocytes) in the blood vessels. The function of these cells is not known but appears to be critical for survival of the stria.

"Pigment-associated inherited deafness is not restricted to dogs. Similar defects have been reported for mice, mink, pigs, horses, cattle, cats, and humans. Deafness in blue-eyed white cats is common and is known to be passed on as an autosomal dominant defect. Blue eyes, resulting from absence of pigment in the iris, is common with pigment-associated deafness but is not, in and of itself, an indication of deafness or the presence of a deafness gene."

SHOULD CONGENITALLY DEAF DOGS BE BRED?

Absolutely not. Based on Dr. Strain's research, it can be confirmed that they will pass on the genetic defect that causes deafness to their offspring. That is why it is a must that all owners of deaf dogs spay or neuter their dogs. It is sad but true that many breeders continue to breed dogs that they know have a history of giving birth to deaf pups, or actually breed dogs who are deaf!

In his *Discussion on Dalmatian Deafness* on his website, Dr. Strain explains, "From data I have collected on hearing tests of about 4,500 Dalmatians, if only one parent is unilaterally deaf [deaf in one ear], the probability nearly DOUBLES that any offspring will be unilaterally deaf or bilaterally deaf. Eight percent of all Dalmatians are bilaterally deaf and 22% are unilaterally deaf - 30% total with some deafness."

(For his detailed reports on deafness in dogs, visit Dr. Strain's website at: <http://www.lsu.edu/guests/senate/public_html/deaf.htm>.

ARE CONGENITALLY DEAF DOGS BRAIN DAMAGED?

No, they are not. Again, I turn to Dr. Strain's article in the British Veterinary Journal. "It has been shown that the auditory cortex of deaf Dalmatians is grossly reduced in size (Ferrara & Halnan,1983) leading the authors to the suggestion that the origin of deafness in the breed was central rather than peripheral. Although not reported, it is likely that other Central Nervous System (CNS) structures in the auditory pathway were also smaller than in hearing animals. However, it is well known from classical studies that kittens whose eyelids were sealed after birth failed to develop normal CNS visual structures, demonstrating that normal sensory input is necessary for the full maintenance of these structures. The findings in the Dal are undoubtedly a reflection of the same pathology. These CNS changes in deaf dogs have been used to justify euthanasia on the basis of having an 'abnormal' brain, but neurologically the brain function of deaf animals is normal except for the loss of auditory function."

In the Management section of the same paper, Strain gives this summary, "...these animals do not have diminished mental capacities, any more than the average deaf or blind human has diminished mental capacity."

ARE DEAF DOGS MORE AGGRESSIVE THAN HEARING DOGS?

In over two years of research, I have found no statistics that prove they are. I have, however, learned several important contributing factors that have to be considered in the case of an aggressive dog, whether hearing *or* deaf. First, I found that aggressive dogs might have had trauma and abuse in their past. I discovered that the disposition of a dog's breed type can make them more dominant, such as guard dogs. Next, dogs can be predisposed to temperament problems because of their individual blood line. Finally, the lack of socialization in any dog has a very big influence on their attitude toward humans.

Certainly, there are reported incidences of aggressive deaf dogs who bite strangers and family members. Dr. Strain has reported that one of the deaf Dalmatians from his deaf dog colony (used for his research) bit one of his sons and one lunged at his other son. He believes deafness was a major factor. In his *Discussion on Dalmatian Deafness* on the web, he states, "For every story of someone who has successfully raised and owned a [unilateral] deaf dog, there are two or more of people who tried and only got heartbreak and incredible problems as a result. Not all deaf dogs ultimately develop aggressive or anxious personalities, but there is no way to predict which will or will not, and those that do are the ones that attack neighbors or family members."

Trying to discover the actual statistics of deaf dog attacks and bites, I asked Dr. Strain if he would share his figures with me. He admitted that he had not collected numbers and that most of the stories he had about aggression came to him second, third and fourth hand.

I also contacted the president of the Dalmatian Club of America to ask for the club's own statistics on aggression. I assumed they would be a definitive resource for these figures, because their stance to destroy deaf Dal pups is partially based on the "fact" that "deaf dogs become aggressive." But they too admitted that they have no records (even letters) of attacks or bites that they can share. Hearsay, only.

After contact with about 1,000 deaf dog owners, and many dog experts worldwide, I have found only ten actual first hand reports of aggressive deaf dogs (seven Dalmatians, one Old English Sheep Dog, and two English Setters). Please see the Research section in the back of the book for information about contributing to future Deaf Dog research on aggression.

Not all animal experts agree that deaf dogs are aggressive. Ilana Reisner, DVM from the Cornell University Animal Behavior Clinic communicated the following to one of my fellow deaf dog owners, "We see dogs most commonly for aggression toward owners, strangers and other dogs. We have seen thirteen Dalmatians over the past five years, almost all for aggression. None of these dogs have been clinically deaf....occasionally I will help the owner of a deaf dog with suggestions for training, but we have not heard from owners of deaf Dalmatians or any other breed with complaints regarding temperament. As a behaviorist, I can assert confidently that serious behavior problems are a result of genetic predisposition or 'temperament' combined with environment (learning); if I were presented with a deaf, aggressive dog, I would presume this aggressiveness would have occurred in the hearing dog as well."

When I posted the question of aggression on the Deaf Dog Newsletter, only four members responded with episodes of aggression and all addressed the behavior responsibly and immediately.

While some owners who adopted their deaf dogs from shelters have discussed minor, initial aggressiveness, they usually report that the dog's fear and anxiety can be overcome with understanding, love and patience.

Lynn Sickenger of Florida, owner of a deaf Dalmatian named Dickens states a popular opinion of deaf dog owners when she says, "There are plenty of hearing dogs out there who are overly aggressive, snappy, hyperactive and out of control. Deaf dogs are only difficult to manage if their masters are unaware of the animal's condition. The barrier of silence is easily crossed with the use of visual signals [communication]. With love and patience, what was mistaken as a vicious animal can become a cooperative, devoted canine companion."

Dog's Today magazine's editor and publisher, Beverly Cuddy told me recently in a phone interview, "Deaf dogs deserve a chance at life. The old wives' tale–deaf equals aggressive–just isn't true. In my whole career in the dog world, I have never come across an aggressive deaf dog, nor have I seen a press report of a deaf dog biting anyone."

Lyndsay sums up this subject very well on the Deaf Dog Web Page when he states, "There is no data on the relative incidence of problem behavior in deaf and hearing Dalmatians [or other breeds]. The Kushti Dalmatian Club in England operates a rescue service for Dalmatians which accepts and places both hearing and deaf Dalmatian orphans. Over the last four years they have placed more than three hundred deaf dogs, and have had to take back less than a half a dozen. The majority of those returned were due to human problems such as death and divorce rather than problems with the dogs. To the best of my knowledge this is by far the largest pool of experience with deaf dogs, and the success rate clearly shows that problems with deaf dogs are the exception rather than the rule; just as is the case with hearing dogs."

WHAT CAN YOU DO TO DISCOURAGE AGGRESSION?

Startling the deaf dog seems to be the most common cause of aggressive behavior: coming up from behind and touching the dog (when he doesn't know you're there), and waking the deaf dog from sleep. Lots of touch when your puppy is young with strong doses of socialization can help prevent this. In the case of an adopted dog who has much to overcome, owners have advised gradual, then increased socialization, and gently touching your dog always in the same place to get their attention (shoulder, hip). See the Socialization section in Chapter Five for more detailed information.

To wake the dog, try any of the following methods: softly blow in the dog's face, touch the dog gently in the same place, put your hand in front of your dog's nose and let your smell wake him. For a while, give a treat every time you wake him. When the startle response begins to diminish, ask visitors to wake the dog with the method you have chosen to use.

One owner I spoke with whose dog has become aggressive after five years has not chosen to euthanise her pet. Instead, she consulted a behaviorist to learn how to deal with the aggression: methods for calming and controlling the dog, a special halter, muzzle and leash for more control of the dog when walking, and when visitors come to the house, the dog is put safely away from the company. While this takes extra time and effort, she loves her dog and he loves the family. Note here that the family has another deaf dog of the same breed who is the same age and has been with the family the same length of time and shows absolutely no signs of aggression.

She ended our conversation by saying that there are many hearing dogs who can begin to exhibit the same aggressive tendencies. Breed, socialization and temperament are key factors in aggression.

I believe a clear perspective can be gained by looking at aggression in all dogs, hearing *and* deaf. It is estimated that at least one million bites from mammals occur each year in North America. Dog bites account for 80-90% of these injuries. I am not able to find a number on deaf dog bites, but how many do you think involve deaf dogs? Fact is, any dog that feels startled, afraid or threatened and/or has endured abuse and abandonment could have aggressive tendencies...not just deaf dogs. And don't forget: there are some breeds who are more genetically and temperamentally aggressive than others.

ARE DEAF DOGS GOOD WITH CHILDREN?

One of my fellow deaf dog owners said it best, "Dogs are good with kids that are good with dogs." And another factor to consider is the breed. Anytime you are contemplating adopting or buying a dog and there are children in your family, check the facts on the breed's basic temperament. Some dogs are better than others with children...hearing or deaf.

My recommended, standard protocol is to first explain to visiting or approaching children (and adults too) that your dog is deaf. Advise them to be calm and still. I explain that deaf dogs hear by watching their movements and if they move fast and wave their arms, it seems like they are yelling to a deaf dog. I always teach the child a sign Spanky is familiar with (usually "good girl" or *toy*) and have them sign to her. Tell them it is best to pet a deaf dog under their head instead of on top of it. The age old advice about putting your hand out (flat with palm up) and letting a dog smell it before you pet it is great advice when reaching to pet any dog.

What did I find in my research about deaf dogs and children? Of the ten cases of aggression or biting that I have on file, half of them involved children under the age of eleven and deaf Dalmatians. I report this only as a cautionary measure. In most cases, Dalmatians, hearing and deaf, live peacefully and happily in families with children.

Dr. Nicholas Dodman, in his book *The Dog Who Loved Too Much*, says of the beloved Dal, "The Disney movie, *101 Dalmatians* popularized the Dalmatian, a dog originally bred in the 1800's for guarding carriages. The Dalmatian's guarding tendencies stem from dominance and protectiveness. The hidden side of their personality is contrary to the expectations of young film-goers who imagine that all dogs of this breed are lovable and friendly, just like their Disney caricatures."

He goes on to say, "I would strongly suggest that anybody who is about to purchase a new dog think seriously about the temperament and manageability of the breed they are planning to acquire." As resources, he recommends *Harper's Guide to Dogs*, edited by Roger Caras, or *Selecting a Puppy*, by Drs. Ben and Lynette Hart. As an owner, you will find Dr. Dodman's book will give you incredible insight into the psychology of dogs, important knowledge for a dog owner, hearing or deaf.

WHAT CAUSES ACQUIRED DEAFNESS?

Deafness can be caused by several things, including illnesses. Chronic ear infections are known to be a leading cause of deafness in dogs. Some dogs develop tumors or polyps which can cause deafness, though this problem can often be remedied with surgery...and believe it or not, if the hearing is restored, but diminished, the dog can be fitted with a hearing aid!

Dr. Strain reports that acquired deafness can also result from any of a large number of drugs and chemicals which directly or indirectly destroy cochlear hair cells. He states, "The effects are dose-dependent and in rare cases reversible. The most commonly recognized ototoxic drugs are the aminoglycoside antibiotics." And then, of course, there can be hearing loss in hunting dogs and pets, in general, as they grow older.

CAN DOGS WHO LOSE THEIR HEARING LIVE FULL LIVES?

Sure they can. Your dog has already learned the rules and routines of home, has observed your body language for years, and each of you knows what to expect of the other. You must simply learn to sign to communicate, learn to wake your dog gently, be a bit more patient, socialize your dog, and take safety measures to guard against your pet being hit by a car. The same communication and training information in this book applies to dogs who acquired their deafness as those dogs who were born deaf.

Dog Breeds With Reported Congenital Deafness 6/97 (Breeds in bold type = relative high prevalence)

Akita

American Eskimo

American Staffordshire Terrier

Australian Cattle Dog

Australian Shepherd

Beagle

Bichon Frise

Border Collie

Boston Terrier

Boxer

Bulldog

Bull Terrier

Cardigan Welsh Corgi

Catahoula Leopard Dog

Cavalier King Charles Spaniel

Chow Chow

Cocker Spaniel

Collie

Dalmatian

Dappled Dachshund

Doberman Pinscher

Dogo Argentino

English Bulldog

English Cocker Spaniel

English Setter

Foxhound

Fox Terrier

French Bulldog

German Shepherd

Great Dane

Great Pyrenees

Ibizan Hound

Italian Greyhound

Jack Russell Terrier

Kuvasz

Labrador Retriever

Maltese

Miniature Pinscher

Miniature Poodle

mongrel

Norwegian Dunkerhound

Old English Sheepdog

Papillon

Pit Bull Terrier

Pointer

Puli

Rhodesian Ridgeback

Rottweiler

Saint Bernard

Schnauzer

Scottish Terrier

Sealyham Terrier

Shetland Sheepdog

Shropshire Terrier

Siberian Husky

Soft Coated Wheaten Terrier

Springer Spaniel

Sussex Spaniel

Tibetan Terrier

Toy Poodle

Walker American Foxhound

West Highland White Terrier

Whippet

Yorkshire Terrier

NOTE: This list provided by Dr. George Strain.
NOTE FROM SUSAN COPE BECKER: When I began my research over two years ago, this chart listed 46 breeds. Today there are 64.

The BAER test confirmed that Spanky has no degree of hearing in either ear. Two flat lines moved across the page showing no response to the sounds introduced during the test.

CHAPTER THREE

Testing Your Dog
For Deafness

How did you know she was deaf? This is a question I have answered many times over the last two years. And while I picked up on Spanky's inability to hear within about four hours, that is not necessarily the norm. Again, I believe one reason I noticed so quickly is because I am familiar with the Boston breed. Another reason is that I was with her all day.

But back to the question, how did I know? When I left the room, she would scream at the top of her lungs. When I called from the room I was in, she didn't come looking for me. When I walked into the room and spoke to her to let her know I had returned, she didn't turn to see me. When she bit me, she did not let go when I cried out. When she had her back to me playing with a toy, I couldn't get her to turn to me when I called.

HEARING TEST TO DO AT HOME

I devised several ways to test her and some fooled me. Basically, they were the same "tests" my veterinarian used to observe her response to sound. This is a list of a "Do-It-Yourself Hearing Tests" you can try at home.

- Have someone hold the dog away from you. Squeeze a squeaky toy behind the dog. Be sure the air that is squeezed from the toy does not reach the dog. When I tried this one the first time, the air alerted her to something behind her and she turned. I was delighted until I realized what had happened.

- Repeat the same posture as above. Clap your hands. Whistle.
- Try these same noises when the dog is sleeping. Do not stand too close to the dog, because, as I mentioned before, the air movement can wake the dog.
- Have someone hold the dog away from you and turn on the vacuum cleaner or another loud appliance. Don't be fooled if the machine creates a vibration on the floor. The deaf dog is very keen to vibration.
- Purchase a dog whistle and blow it in the same room as the dog.

After these tests, I was convinced that Spanky could not hear. We visited the veterinarian where he repeated the same "tests" and pronounced her deaf. He then inquired at the University of Tennessee about further testing and asked for some basic training instruction for me. When I called to speak with Dr. Sims, I was told about the BAER test. I scheduled one right away even though I was fairly certain that Spanky was deaf.

Why? I noticed her moving her head suddenly when the kids ran out to the playground at the neighboring school. Or I observed her jumping up from a sound sleep minutes after someone came into the house. She turned and looked when someone entered the room where she was laying on the floor with a chew toy. She seemed so alert. I guess at that point I was desperately hoping that she could maybe, just maybe, hear something.

WHAT IS THE BAER TEST?

Dr. Michael Sims, Ph.D., Physiologist at the University of Tennessee School of Veterinary Medicine explains, "The brainstem auditory evoked response (BAER, pronounced "bear") procedure consists of using computers to record time-averaged electrical activity from the brain in response to repetitive sound stimulation. Such procedures are necessary because like animals, not all human beings are able to communicate effectively. This is especially true for human infants, many of whom are evaluated for auditory function within the first postnatal week.

"The most common application of this technique was to assist in the diagnosis of cochlear agenesis, a hereditary types of deafness that was beginning to appear in purebred dogs at an alarming rate.

"The cochlea is the device in the inner ear that converts the sound

36

waves to electrochemical impulses that travel to the brain. If the cochlea is not functional, then the animal is totally deaf on the side of dysfunction. Trying to determine if an animal hears sounds is frustrating because of its response to visual cues and vibrations associated with airborne sounds. The latter is sometimes referred to as extracochlear hearing and is particularly well-developed in some species."

Dr. Sims advises, "Unilateral deafness [deaf in one ear] in puppies is practically impossible to detect on the basis of behavioral responses to sound and even difficult in adults. Suspected bilateral deafness should be confirmed electrodiagnostically, and all purebred pups with a high breed-specific occurrence of deafness should be tested. In dogs, the BAER is an excellent means of identifying totally deaf or unilaterally deaf puppies."

HOW IS THE BAER TEST PERFORMED AND IS IT PAINFUL?

Puppies can be effectively BAER tested after they reach six to eight weeks of age. Earlier testing can give false results because ear canals remain closed for several weeks after birth.

To perform the test, electrodes are placed under the skin on the dog's head, and are connected to a computer that introduces a series of clicks that are directed into the ear with an earphone. The computer measures the brainstem auditory response and a print out shows the actual recorded waveforms. Lines jumping up and down reflect hearing. Flat lines show no hearing.

Dr. Strain explains the BAER test on his web site. I will quote a brief description of the test. "The response is collected with a special computer through extremely small electrodes placed under the skin of the scalp; one in front of each ear, on at the top of the head, and one between and behind the eyes. It is rare for a dog to show any evidence of pain from the placement of the electrodes–if anything the dog objects to the gentle restraint and the irritation of wires hanging in front of its face. Sedation or anesthesia are usually not necessary unless the dog becomes extremely agitated, which can usually be avoided with patient and gentle handling."

The BAER test confirmed that Spanky has no degree of hearing in either ear. Two flat lines moved across the page showing no response to the sounds introduced during the test.

While some dogs I have heard of go through the test with no stress or fear, Spanky was terrified. She indeed became "severely agitated" and as a result was sedated. Perhaps it is because I was not allowed to be with her during the test. But whatever the reason, this experience has made going to the veterinarian traumatic since then. She doesn't want anyone looking into her ears or holding her in place on an examination table.

In the big scheme of things, it really didn't matter if she could hear a little or not, and I feel like I had the test done more for myself than for Spanky. I am not advising against the BAER test, but if I had it to do over, I would not have put her through it.

BAER TESTING SITES

This list provided is a combination of a list from the Deaf Dog Mailing List and Dr. George Strain's BAER site list (updated 3/98). Dr. Strain's note follows: This list is not an endorsement of the abilities of the individuals listed and I assume no liability by providing it. This also is not a guarantee that the following sites are still active. I would greatly appreciate being informed of inactive sites as well as new ones not currently listed.

Inside of the United States

Dr. A. Edward Marshall
Auburn University
Department of Anatomy & Histology
College of Veterinary Medicine
Auburn University, AL 36849-5518
205-844-6741

Dr. Janet Steiss
Scott - Richey Research Center
Auburn University College of
    Veterinary Medicine
Auburn University, AL 36849
334-844-5564
steisje@vetmed.auburn.edu

Dr. Donald Levesque
Veterinary Neurological Center
4202 East Raymond Street
Phoenix, AZ 85040-1935
DCLNEURO@aol.com

Dr. Randall C. Longshore
Veterinary Neurological Center
4202 E. Raymond St.
Phoenix, AZ 85040-1935
602-437-1488, fax 602-437-5425

D. Collette Williams
UC Davis Vet School
Davis, CA
916-752-1355
916-752-1393

Dr. Mark Wright
Plaza Veterinary Clinic
7340 Firestone Blvd. Unit 117
Downey, CA 90241
310-928-2234

Dr. Candace A. Sousa
Animal Dermatology Clinic
5701 H Street
Sacramento, CA 95819
916-451-6445

Dr. Richard Hoskins
Redwood Veterinary Clinic
Santa Rosa, CA
707-542-4012

Susan Hurt, Audiologist
2965 Tuxedo Place
Santa Rosa, CA 95405
BAER testing for Dr. Poplin, DVM

Dr. Thomas Schubert
Old River Veterinary Hospital
520 West 11th St.
Tracy, CA 95376
209-835-5166

Michael Ericson, DVM
25 Adeline Drive
Walnut Creek, CA 94596
510-930-0383
510-934-6596
FAX 510-930-7941

Dr. Stephen Hanson
Southern California Surgical Group
17672 Cowan Ave., Suite A-100
Irvine, CA 92614
714-833-9020
FAX 714-833-7530

Dr. Steve Coulter
Rocky Mountain Veterinary
   Neurological Associates
1819 West Prospect
Fort Collins, CO 80526
303-935-9346

Dr. Paul Cuddon
Colorado State University
CVMBS-VTH, Clinical Sciences
300 West Drake Road
Ft. Collins, CO 80523
970-491-4461
FAX 970-491-1275
pcuddon@vagus.vth.colostate.edu

Dr. Patricia J. Luttgen
Neurological Center for Animals
7261 W. Hampden Ave.
Lakewood, CO 80227-5305
303-989-4656
FAX 303-989-4666
PJLNEURO@aol.com

Dr. Mary O. Smith
Assistant Professor of Neurology
Colorado State University
Veterinary Teaching Hospital
300 West Drake Road
Ft. Collins, CO 80523
303-491-0316
FAX 970-491-1275
msmith@vagus.vth.colostate.edu

Dr. Pierre Bichsel
Animal Emergency & Referral Center
3984 S. US Highway 1
Fort Pierce, FL 54982
561-466-3441

Dr. Julie Blackmore
2229 S. Kannet Highway
Stuart, FL 34994
407-286-2338

Dr. Andy Hopkins
North Florida Neurology
1015 SE Lake Lane
Keystone Heights, FL 32656
904-269-7070
FAX 352-473-5580

Dr. Gillian Irving
6209 Walsh Lane
Tampa, FL 33625
813-968-6175

Dr. Glen Mayer
Abell Animal Hospital
6032 Northwest Highway
Chicago, IL 60631
312-631-6727

Dr. Karen Kline
Iowa State University
Veterinary Clinical Services
College of Veterinary Medicine
Ames, IA 50010
515-294-4900
FAX 515-294-9281
kkline@cvmoi.vm.iastate.edu

Dr. Phil March
Purdue University, School of
    Veterinary Medicine
Department of Clinical Sciences
1248 Lynn Hall
West Lafayette, IN 47907
317-494-9333
FAX 317-496-1166

Dr. N. Sidney Remmele
Remmele Animal Clinic
2060 Idle Hour Center
Lexington, KY 40502
606-269-0000, fax 606-269-0022

Dr. George Strain
LSU School of Veterinary Medicine
Baton Rouge, LA 70803
504-388-5833
FAX 504-388-5983
strain@.lsu.edu

Larry Gainsburg, DVM
Baltimore Vet Referral Service
1315 Kingsbury Road
Owings Mills, MD 21117
301-363-1373

Dr. Kim Knowles
Tufts University, School of
    Veterinary Medicine
Department of Medicine
200 Westboro Road
North Grafton, MA 01536
508-839-5395, Beeper #5'
FAX 508-839-7922

Dr. Charles Lowrie
Michigan State University
Veterinary Medical Teaching Hospital
East Lansing, MI 48824-1314

Dr. Julie Haas
Michigan Veterinary Specialists
21600 W. Eleven Mile
Southfield, MI 48076
313-354-6660

Dr. S.B. Shelton
Michigan Veterinary Specialists
21600 W. Eleven Mile
Southfield, MI 48076
313-354-6660

Dr. Michael Wolf
Oakland Veterinary Referral Service
1940 S. Telegraph Road
Bloomfield Hills, MI 48302
810-334-6877
FAX 810-334-3693

Dave Jennings, DVM
Mississippi State University
College of Veterinary Medicine,
Drawer V
Mississippi State, MS 39762
601-325-1489

Dr. Dennis O'Brien
University of Missouri
School of Veterinary Medicine
379 East Campus Drive, Room A375
Columbia, MO 65211
573-882-7821
FAX 573-884-5444
obrien@vets.vetmed.missouri.edu

Dr. Susanne Hughes
Colony Park Animal Hospital
3102 Sandy Creek Dr.
Durham, NC 27705
919-489-9156

Dr. Anthony DeCarle
Red Bank Veterinary Hospital
210 Newman Springs Road
Red Bank, NJ 07701

Dr. Edgar Gasteiger
Cornell University
204 Ithaca Road
Ithaca, NY 14850
607-253-3547

Dr. Ellis Loew
Cornell University College of Veterinary
Medicine
Physiology T6-026A
Ithaca, NY 14853
607-253-3484
607-253-3490 Lab

Dr. Richard Joseph
Animal Medical Center - Bobst Hospital
510 East 62nd Street
New York, NY 10021-8383
212-838-8100

Dr. Michael Podell
The Ohio State University
Dept. of Veterinary Clinical
  Services
College of Veterinary Medicine
601 Vernon L. Tharp Street
Columbus, OH 43210
614-688-3792
614-292 0895
podell.1@osu.edu

Dr. James Breazile
Oklahoma State University
College of Veterinary Medicine
Stillwater, OK 74078-0107
405-744-8089

Dr. Robert A. Kroll
Oregon Veterinary Specialty Clinic
4905 S.W. 77th Ave.
Portland, OR 97225
503-292-3001
krollr@ohsu.edu

Larry Martin, Audiologist
Audiology Services
2371 Oakmont Way
Eugene, OR 97401
503-484-4327

Dr. Steven Skinner
Oregon Veterinary Referral Center
4905 S.W. 77th Ave.
Portland, OR 97225
503-292-3001

Dr. Betsy Dayrell-Hart
University of Pennsylvania, Dept. of
Clinical Studies
School of Veterinary Medicine
3900 Delancy Street
Philadelphia, PA 19104-6010
215-898-6473
FAX 215-573-3925
bdh@pobox.upenn.edu

Daniel M. Burnside, VMD
Quakertown Veterinary Clinic
2250 Old Bethlehem Pike
Quakertown, PA 18951
215-536-6245

Dr. Mickey Sims
University of Tennessee
Department of Animal Science
College of Veterinary Medicine
POB 1071
Knoxville, TN 37901-1071
615-974-5820

Dr. Joan Coates
Texas A&M University
College of Veterinary Medicine
Small Animal Medicine and
Surgery
College Station, TX 77843

Dr. Karen Dyer Inzana
Dr. Linda Shell
Virginia-Maryland Regional
College of Veterinary Medicine
Duck Pond Drive
Virginia Tech University
Blacksburg, VA 24061
540-231-4621

Dr. Michael Moore
Washington State University
Veterinary Clinical Sciences
Pullman, WA 99164-6610
509-335-0711
FAX 509-335-0880

Dr. Anne Chauvet
University of Wisconsin
Veterinary Clinic
2015 Linden Drive West
Madison, WI 53706
608-263-7600
FAX 608-265-8020
chauvet@svm.vetmed.wisc.edu

Outside of the United States

Dr. Clive Eger
Murdoch University Veterinary
   Hospital
School of Veterinary Studies
South Street
Murdoch, Perth
Western Australia 6150
Australia
61-09-360-2641
FAX 61-09-310-7495
eger@numbat.murdoch.edu.au

Dr. Richard Malik
University of Sydney
Veterinary Clinical Sciences
B10 - Evelyn Williams
Sydney, NSW 2006
Australia
61 2 9351 3437
FAX 61 2 9351 4261
malik@mail.usyd.edu.au

Dr. Sue Summerlad
University of Queensland
Brisbane, Queensland
Australia
61 7 3365 2110

Dr. Gerold Maier
Gruental 286
A-3400 Klosterneuburg
Vienna
Austria
43 (0) 2243 83869

Dr. Birgit Seitlinger
Audiometrische Ambulanz der
Veterinarmedizinischen Universitat
Institut fur Physiologie
Veterinarplatz 1
A-1210 Wien (Vienna)
Austria
43-1-250 77 - 4501, fax 43-1-250 77 -
4590
8945018@bendomsrv.vu-wien.ac.at

Dr. L. Poncelet
Small Animal Surgery Department
Faculty of Veterinary Medicine
University of Liège
B-4000 Liège (Sart Tilman)
Belgium

Dr. Joanne Parent
University of Guelph
Ontario Veterinary College
Guelph Ontario N1G 2W1
Canada
519-823-8830
FAX 519-767-0311
jparent@ovcnet.uoguelph.ca

Dr. Susan Cochrane
Morningside Animal Clinic
4560 Kingston Road
Scarborough Ontario M1E 2P2
Canada
416-284-9205
FAX 416-287-3642

Dr. Andrea Quesnel
Université de Montreal
Faculte de Medecine Vet.
3200 Rue Sciotte, C. P. 5000
St. Hyacinthe, Quebec J2T 2L6
Canada
514-778-8111
FAX 514-778-8110

Gillian D. Muir, DVM, Phd
University of Saskatchewan
Veterinary Physiological Sciences
52 Campus Drive
Saskatoon, SK S7N B54 Canada
306-966-7353
FAX 306-966-7376
muir@admin3.usask.ca

Dr. Agnes Delauche
Centre for Small Animal Studies
Animal Health Trust, PO Box 5
Newmarket, Suffolk CB8 8JH
England
+44 (0) 1638 661111
FAX +44 (0) 1638 555600

Mr. Geoff Skerritt
Church Farm Veterinary Clinic
Neston Road, South Wirral
Liverpool, Merseyside L64 2TL
England
0151 327 1855

Faculty of Veterinary Medicine
Library of Veterinary Medicine
P.O. Box 57
00014 University of Helsinki
Finland
FAX. 358-9-70849-799)
kirjasto@vetmed.fi

Dr. Suvi Pohjola-Stenroos
Clinivet Oy
Lansikaari 2 A
08500 Lohja as
Finland
fax 358-19-383 473
clinivet@sci.fi

Dr. N. Dykshoorn
Utrechtseweg 50
3704 HE Zeist
Netherlands
030 6954264, fax 030 6950004

Dr. Anjop J. Venker-van Haagen
Faculty of Veterinary Medicine
Department of Clinical Sciences of
Companion Animals
PO Box 80.154
3508 TD Utrecht
Netherlands
A.J.VenkervH@ukg.dgk.ruu.nl

Dr. Antony Goodhead
Onderstepoort Veterinary Hospital
University of Pretoria
Onderstopoort, 0110
South Africa
JAEH@op1.up.ac.za

Dr. Remo Lobetti
Department of Medicine
Faculty of Veterinary Science
University of Pretoria
Private Bag X04
Onderstepoort, 0110
South Africa
27-12-5298000, Fax: 27-12-5298308
genees5@op1.up.ac.za

Dr. Lennart Sjostrom
Regiondjursjukhuset i Strmsholm
Strmsholm Referral Animal Hospital
S-730 40 Kolback
Sweden
+46 - 22043200
lennart.sjostrom@vasteras.mail.telia.com

PLEASE NOTE:
If you have an update for this list, please send the information to me for my revisions and I will also forward it to Dr. Strain.

...a dog who has moved into advanced training for police work, hunting, hearing dog work with deaf owners, combat duty, or television and movies is trained to hand signs. Teaching a dog hand signs is not as unusual as you might think.

CHAPTER FOUR

How To Communicate
With Your Deaf Dog

Hand signs are the "words" you use to communicate with your deaf dog. You will probably find yourself using a combination of American Sign Language (ASL), Standard Obedience signs and signs that you invent. Any and all of these are okay. What's important is that you and your dog understand each other, and that you use the signs you choose consistently. The advantages to American Sign Language are: it is more widely used, you will find that more people can "talk" to your dog; ASL is illustrated so they are easier to learn and share with friends and family; an inexpensive paperback of ASL is available at most book stores. One very important tip: always try to simplify the sign to one hand because at times you will find yourself unable to use two hands.

Using hand signs may feel a bit awkward to you at first, and you may forget them (another reason to keep a copy handy). But the more you use them, the quicker you and your dog will learn and remember them.

DO DOGS UNDERSTAND SIGN LANGUAGE?

Yes. Dogs naturally communicate with body language, posturing, and subtle signals. And don't forget, a dog who has moved into advanced training for police work, hunting, hearing dog work with deaf owners, combat duty, or television and movies is trained to hand signs. Teaching a dog hand signs is not as unusual as you might think.

Remember, as you sign to your dog, talk aloud also. Your facial expressions and body language will help communicate the message, positive or negative. Be animated and expressive as you sign. Sign clearly and consistently. For instance, when you use the sign for *down, stop* or *no,* sign firmly with authority. You might have to sign it two or three times in rapid succession to show you mean business (especially *no*). For instance, if I am working and Spanky is being persistent about playing, it takes three rapid *no* signs. When I do this, she usually sighs loudly and leaves me alone. Some owners shake their index finger in warning before signing *no* and sometimes, this is enough.

HOW DO I TEACH A SIGN TO MY DOG?

Repetition and patience. Begin with the basics. With Spanky, I began with *no, good, sit* and *stay.* After your dog gets the hang of watching your hands for communication, expand.

To teach a sign to your dog, such as *ball,* hold the ball in your hand and show it to your dog. Tuck it under your arm and sign *ball.* Repeat two or three times. Throw it and when your dog returns it, repeat the sign again. Your dog will catch on quickly.

When I taught Spanky *car,* I signed *car* before we went out, and after we were in the car I signed it again. Sign *walk* before and during your walk. It's just like teaching a word to your dog.

You say it when you do it and you say it a lot. Again, repetition is the key to teaching a new sign to your dog...repetition and patience.

WHEN SHOULD I USE SIGNS WITH MY DOG?

Sign to your dog anytime you would normally "talk" to your dog to give a command, to reassure or praise. If it is *no, stay, stop* that you want to communicate, sign it and say it aloud. If it is *go get your ball,* sign *go* and *ball* and say, "Go get your ball." When you are preparing to feed your dog, sign *bite* frequently (using your fingers as if you were holding something, act like you are putting it in your mouth).

HOW DO I USE SIGNS DURING TRAINING?

Begin with the basics, just as if you were training a hearing dog. Start with *sit* and *lie down.* Spend about 10 to 15 minutes on *sit,* pushing your dogs rump down to a sitting position, rewarding with a treat and/or touch. Advance to *down* in the same session. Work with your dog on these two obedience commands 10 to 15 minutes two-three times each day. If you've never trained a dog (hearing or deaf) by all means consult a good training book, or better yet, sign up for a basic obedience class with a trainer in your area. (see *Sit, Lie Down and Stay* in Chapter 5)

HOW CAN I TEACH OTHERS TO COMMUNICATE WITH MY DOG?

I highly recommend photocopying the basic signs you use with your dog and showing them to frequent visitors to your home to enable them to communicate with your dog too. Post a copy of them in your kitchen or a high traffic area in your home where visitors can easily consult them.

When you observe someone trying to say *no* or *stop* or *down* by pushing your dog away, demonstrate and encourage them to use the proper sign. When you find an obedience class, be sure to let the trainer know that you will provide them with the signs that will be needed for the basics. Offer to let them read this book before the class begins. Many trainers are willing to train a deaf dog, but never have. This book will offer them added information they need to couple with their own training skills for great success.

HOW CAN I LEARN MORE SIGNS TO TEACH MY DOG?

To expand your vocabulary and your dog's, use a pocket-sized version of American Sign Language. It is inexpensive and invaluable. Other signs you might need are *quiet* (the sign your librarian used), *finished* (act as if you are shaking something off of your hands) and *door* (I hold both hands open chest high, palms facing out with thumb sides together and pull them apart as if they are opening to let Spanky know someone is at the door). It just depends on how far you want to go with your dog's vocabulary. Some dogs who are six to seven years old know between 40 and 50 signs!

Other ASL signs you will find useful: *outside* or *toilet, sleep* or *bed*. As you find the need for a new word, look it up, learn it and teach it to your dog.

The following illustrated signs are constants in Spanky's vocabulary. After the illustrations, you will find written description of several (some the same word with different sign) that are used by fellow deaf dog owners. None of these are right or wrong. Just choose the one that works best for you and be sure that all family members and friends know the basics.

BALL

Curve your hands with fingertips touching, forming a ball.
Memory Tip: The round shape identifies a ball.
American Sign Language

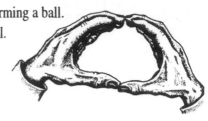

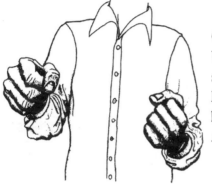

CAR

Use both hands to move an imaginary steering wheel.
Memory Tip: Hands are in the position of holding a steering wheel.
American Sign Language

COME

Hold hand flat in front of you and pull to your chest.
Standard Obedience Sign

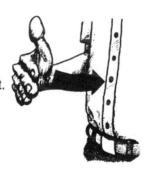

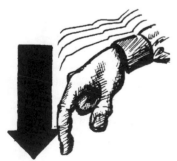

DOWN/when jumping or on furniture

Point the right index finger down and move it down slightly.
Memory Tip: Finger pointing downward.
American Sign Language

GO/also used for FETCH
Point in the direction you want your dog to go,
or in the direction that you have thrown their toy.
I use this and then "ball" to tell
Spanky to go get her ball.
Invented Sign

GOOD GIRL/GOOD
NOTE: I use the sign for "girl" to say "good girl" to
Spanky. Right thumb is moved down the jaw line
from ear to chin.
I also clap my hands to sign "good" to her. It is
very enthusiastic praise. Some use "thumbs up."
American Sign Language

LIE DOWN
Use right hand stretched flat with palm down.
Move hand down toward floor.
Standard Obedience Sign

NO

Bring the right thumb, index and middle fingers together. Some owners shake a pointing finger as a warning before signing *no*.

Memory Tip: A combination of the signs for N and O.

American Sign Language

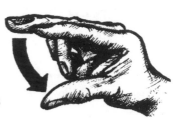

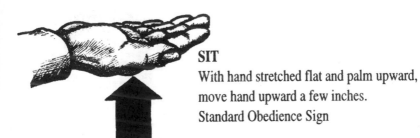

SIT

With hand stretched flat and palm upward, move hand upward a few inches.

Standard Obedience Sign

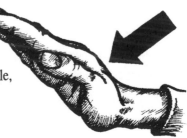

STAY

With hand stretched flat and held at an angle, move forward a few inches.

Standard Obedience Sign

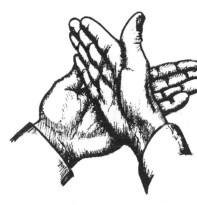

STOP

With both hands stretched flat, hold the
left hand flat in front of you and
chop it with your right hand.
Memory Tip: Suggest a barrier that
would stop progress.
American Sign Language

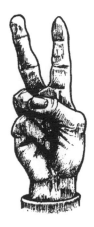

TOY

Raise the index and middle fingers and wiggle like rabbit ears.
Memory Tip: As a pup, Spanky's favorite toy was a stuffed
bunny, so I indicated the ears with my fingers.
Invented Sign

WALK

Use index and middle fingers and move as if they
are walking in the air.
Memory Tip: Do as if fingers are walking
on a surface.
Invented Sign

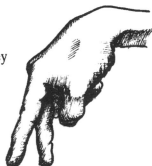

53

MORE HAND SIGNS

These signs and comments are from my fellow deaf dog owners and me. You might find some of these more natural for you to use than the illustrated signs preceding this section. Remember, however, that the sign you choose to use should be used consistently.

BAD

• Spanky knows the ASL sign for bad. Hold your hand facing outward and bend the fingers over toward the palm like claws.

COME

• A universal sign for people in dog language for *come* is to raise a hand. Every time the dog starts towards you, for whatever reason, raise your hand. Pretty soon, your pup realizes that when you raise your hand, and he comes, he's done something good, and gets praised.

• When I am moving to another room or location inside or outside the house, I have a more relaxed way of signaling come to Spanky. I hold my hand palm up, fingers together and bend my fingers back and forth. This is more of an invitation that a command.

• Motion index finger toward you (not an easy one to see from a distance).

• Wave arms over head back and forth (good for long distances).

• Hands slapping your knees.

DOOR

• Hold both hands open, palms flat and facing outward, and hold thumb sides together. Pull them apart as if they are opening. Use this sign to say that someone is at the door or someone has come in the house. Spanky always perks up her ears, gives a bark or two and heads for the door anxiously anticipating attention and play time from whoever has arrived.

DROP

• Clench your fist with finger-side facing the ground. Open your fingers as if you are dropping something.

EAT
• Hold your fingers together as if you have a bite of something in your hand and raise it to your lips. When I put Spanky's food out (if she is not already underfoot), I go find her and sign "eat." She comes running.

FINISHED/THAT'S ALL
• Wipe your right hand (palm down) over your left hand (palm up) as if you are brushing something off of your hands.

GOOD/GOOD JOB/GOOD DOG
• Place the fingers of the right flat over your lips, hold your the left hand flat and facing up about waist-high; now move the right hand from the lips downward into the left hand.
• When Spanky fetches a toy, I clap as she returns to me. I also use this sign when she is good. In a sense, it is also my sign for *yes*.
• Some owners use the thumbs up sign to signal good.
• Don't forget to smile and shake your head *yes*.
• Fingertips on right hand touching lips then move downward with hand open.

HELLO
• Wave to your dog. When Spanky comes into the room when she rouses herself from bed in the morning (she always sleeps in), we wave and smile at her in welcome.
• When I see her across the room or lawn, I wave to her. I consider this as calling her name.

I'LL BE BACK OR JUST A MINUTE
• I hold up one finger as if to say, "Just a minute. I'll be back." I use this when I am leaving her at home, or when I leave her in the car (when it's cool enough for her to ride with me) to let her know I'll be right back. This also seems to work when she is impatient about getting something right away.

LOOK AT ME
• Raise your hand and position it beside your eyes.
• To signal Spanky, I point at both eyes at the same time with my index and middle fingers forked.

OKAY

• Thumbs up. Make a fist with your thumb pointing upward. This sign is used to reassure your dog that everything is fine and to be calm.

• Make a circle by touching your thumb to your index finger holding the other three fingers together. A typical A-okay sign.

OUTSIDE

• Roll both hands over each other in front of torso to sign, "Do you want to go outside?"

NO

• Point a shaking finger.

• A very serious *no* is thumb and fingers (the *no* sign) to "snap" the dog's nose.

• Often to show Spanky that I mean business, I use the chopping sign for *stop* (see illustrated signs) several times and sign *no* several times. The chopping *stop* sign is a much stronger looking sign and really gets her attention.

• Shake head back and forth.

• Flat hand, palm down, moving straight across in front of you

QUIET/CALM DOWN

• Use the sign most commonly used for "shhhh" by placing your index finger over your lips like a librarian.

SIGNING YOUR DOG'S NAME

• Some owners sign their dog's name by using the ASL sign for the first letter of the dog's name and either holding it in front of them or tapping their shoulder or chest with it.

• Another owner holds the letter sign for their female dog at the right side of the chin, and for their male dog beside their right eyebrow.

SIGNING NAMES OF FAMILY MEMBERS OR COMPANION DOGS

• Choose a letter from the person or dogs name that is obvious. For instance, to signal my son's dog, Jazz, I use the letter *j* (little finger draws the letter j in the air). When I sign *j* and *door*, Spanky knows Jazz has arrived. Make up a sign if you choose, but again, use the signs consistently.

56

SIT

• ASL sign for sit is to place index and middle fingers of the right hand over the same two fingers of the left hand and move them downward.

Spanky also knows *cows* (I make horns on my head with my two index fingers). I use this sign when we are headed to our cabin in the mountains because a large herd of cows grazes in the field below us and she loves sitting in a chair, front paws on the porch railing watching them move about. I sign *T* the way a football referee (making a *T* with both hands flat) to tell her we are packing the car to go to Tennessee. She knows several signs for friends: *n* for Anne, an invented sign for Granny, fist closed with fingers opening suddenly and upward for her Pop, and *m* for Mary who comes to our home every day to run our office. Spanky also knows the sign for *tree* which tells her we will walk in the woods.

Be creative. When you have a significant word you want to teach your dog that you communicate often, invent a sign (these signs usually come naturally) or look it up in your pocket version of American Sign Language. They will catch on very quickly when you use it consistently and associate it with the object, place or person.

Training the deaf dog is the same as training a hearing dog with the exception of using signs as signals rather than spoken words.

CHAPTER FIVE

Deaf Dog Traits, Training and Safety Tips

Training a deaf dog is basically the same as training a hearing dog. If you have specific training problems or questions, consult any training book that appeals to you or works with your philosophy. I believe the best thing I ever did for Spanky's training was to sign up for a basic obedience class. Many owners go on to higher training and have also reported that agility training greatly improved their dog's confidence and their bond as dog and master.

Training a dog–hearing or deaf– can be frustrating. A dog's attention span is like a child's. The older the child, the longer the attention span. Be patient. Go slow. Above all else, don't lose your temper. If your dog is not in the mood or is too distracted, don't force the issue. Take a break and come back to it. And work only in ten or fifteen minute sessions two or three times a day.

Lyndsay Patten, who established the Deaf Dog Web Page, gives the following tips, "You have to use hand signals rather than verbal commands; it means you need an alternative method for getting and keeping your dog's attention; and it means you'll need to find a substitute for the verbal praise and feedback which are components of most canine training programs." Hopefully, this chapter and the preceding chapter on hand signs will offer you many options to meet these challenges.

An alphabetized list of many tips and techniques follows. They are used by my fellow deaf dog owners and myself. Read them all and use what works best for you and your dog.

ATTENTION

How can you communicate if your dog isn't looking at you? You can't. That's why there are several ways of getting your deaf dog's attention. You will find that the more you communicate with your dog, the more you work with your dog, the more your dog will be attuned to you and your movements and signals. When working with your dog to teach him attention, try to work in an area with as few distractions as possible. Increase distractions as the training continues so your dog learns to watch you and obey you in all conditions. In the beginning, always treat when your dog gives you eye contact.

• Raise your hand and position it beside your eye. Verbalize *watch me*. When your dog gives you eye contact, reward with a treat. Note: I use index and middle finger pointing at my eyes (it makes it easy to hold a treat between thumb and ring finger).
• Bump the floor with your foot or hand.
• Turn a flashlight off and on. (Many deaf dogs like to play with the flashlight beam. It seems to be a lot of fun for dog and owner alike.)
• Some folks use a laser light. Because of it's intensity, it can be used during the day and the beam can be directed to shine on something that is within your dog's vision such as the wall, floor or furniture.
• Waving your arm because their peripheral vision catches the motion.
• If you are in a closed room, clap or shout loudly. Sometimes the sound waves will cause the dog to become alert and look for you.
• Stick little strips of jerky between your lips and when your dog looks at you, let him have it.
• One owner would fill her cheeks with tiny bites of hot dog and when her dog looked at her, she would blow one out for the dog as a reward.
• Fill your pockets with treats and when your dog looks at you, give him a treat.
• One trainer advises making small, lightweight bean bags and tossing them at your dog. Some of the owners I heard discuss this said their dogs thought they were to play with. I have often tossed a toy into Spanky's field of vision to get her to turn to me.

• Electric or Shock Collars are not used by most deaf dog owners, but one owner who uses one reported, "The lowest level of stimulation on his collar is no worse than the amount of electrical stimulation used in physical therapy (it actually feels kind of good, speaking from personal experience). My dog is learning very quickly that the little tingle means that he'll get a treat if he turns and looks at me for a hand signal. It's giving him a greater range of freedom."
• If your dog is outside at night and you want to call him in, turn your porch light off and on rapidly.
• If on leash, jiggle the leash gently.
• See the Collars section of this chapter for information on vibrating collars.

BARKING

It amazes me that people ask so often if Spanky can bark since she is deaf. Can she bark! She barks for longer periods than normal because she can't hear herself. She also makes high pitched barking sounds and whines. Keep in mind that while this doesn't bother her, it drives the rest of us crazy. I believe that because deaf dogs are so visually oriented, they see things in a very intense manner. For instance, Spanky barks at reflections in the windows, leaves blowing on the trees and objects placed in unusual places (a box delivered by UPS will really upset her).

• Sign *no* and *quiet* to your dog. Distract with a toy or an invitation to go to another part of the house.
• Spray your dog with a stream of water from a squirt bottle or water pistol. Then sign *no* and *quiet* to your dog.
• According to one owner, if the deaf dog is an excessive barker, and some are, the Radio Fence Systems bark control collar (or an equivalent product) works well and does not associate the owner with the punishment (a very mild electric shock–if this causes you to wince, try it on yourself first).

BASIC OBEDIENCE

Find a trainer that will take you in a basic obedience class, and/or consult a training book. Use standard obedience signs, American Sign Language signs, and invented signs. Give your trainer a copy of the signs in this book and/or the signs you use with your dog. If you cannot find a trainer to work with, buy a good training manual and follow the basic instructions for teaching: *sit, stay, heel,* and *lie down.* You will find obedience hand signs in some dog training books. (See Sit, Lie Down and Stay in this chapter)

BITING AND MOUTHING

When Spanky nipped or bit at me as a puppy, I used the thumb and two fingers as I signed *no* to lightly pinch her nose. This was not pleasant (although it did not hurt her). Mouthing and biting are behaviors that must be addressed as soon as they occur.

• To curb unwanted biting, fold the dog's lip under one of his teeth and press when your dog bites or nips you. Then sign *no.*
• Clamp your dog's nose and mouth shut, stare him down and sign *no.*
• When your dog is mouthing, stop playing. One owner shared this observation: when puppies play and one puppy bites too hard, the other will stop playing and leave the biting puppy.
• If your dog takes your hand or arm into his mouth, go limp and show by facial expression you are hurt. A gradual process but effective.

CHILDREN INTERACTING WITH DEAF DOGS

I have found that very young children can intimidate and scare Spanky without meaning to. Because the deaf dog watches your every move for signs and for body language, a child who is flailing their arms, darting and jumping around must seem like a screaming, possibly threatening, confusing thing. I have found Spanky gets along fine with children 7 years old and up. The younger ones scare her and she usually makes herself scarce when they are on the scene. (Also see the question on children and deaf dogs on page 30.)

• The moment company arrives have your dog sit and stay and explain to the children and adults alike that your dog is deaf and that it is very easy to frighten her with sudden and excessive movements.
• If they are bigger than your dog, teach them to lean over slightly, extend their hand palm up for the dog to sniff, and then to pet the dog under its chin.
• Teach the child the sign *toy* or *ball* and have a brief play session. This always endears anybody to Spanky...and Spanky to them.
•Tell them never to touch or approach your dog if she is sleeping.

62

CLICKER TRAINING

While I am not familiar with this method and do not use it, many of the Deaf Dog Mailing List members do, and they swear by it. This method is often used to train dolphins, killer whales, and other sea animals. The clicker is the secondary reinforcer and the treat is the primary. The clicker allows you to communicate "that's right" to the dog instantly. The other thing it does is prompt the dog to be creative. One of the newsletter members stated, "I cannot say enough good things about this training method. It is fun for the dog, fun for the trainer, and gives the dog a certain independence in selecting behaviors to perform."

• One mailing list member recommends *Don't Shoot the Dog* and *Lads Before the Wind* both by Karen Pryor.
• The following can be used as clicker substitutes when clicker training a deaf dog: a flashlight or laser light, the hand sign for *click*, a thumbs up signal.

COLLARS

The topic of collars is important with leash training for dogs that pull on the leash. Check the section *Leash Training/Pulling* in this chapter for specific recommendations from deaf dog owners.

Many of us have wished for a vibrating collar for our deaf dogs. While many companies and even deaf dog owners have talked about manufacturing a vibrating collar, to date one is not available for sale. The company who began design and development on the project in 1997, abandoned the project several months later. Perhaps the following is the best solution at the moment.

• Make your own vibrating collar. This message was posted on the Deaf Dog Mailing List by a veterinarian student who owns a deaf and blind dog: "We made a vibrating collar from a radio controlled car. The actual motor from the car is encased in a plastic film case that I sewed to her collar, along with the antenna. When you push the remote that would normally make the car run, the motor spins and causes a vibration on her neck. It's fairly rough in design, but does work. The range of the device is limited, but it has been sufficient to test and see whether positive enforcement and a vibrating collar might work for training and communicating with deaf dogs."

COME

• Try playing a game of tag with your dog to teach come. Most dogs are programmed to follow a leader, so if you run away from the dog he will run after you. Stop. When the dog catches up, reward with a treat.

COMPANION DOG

Spanky lived her first year as an "only child." When I moved to Cincinnati with Ethan, she got a new stepsister, a seven year old German Short Hair named Joy. Joy was not very excited about giving up her "only child" status, but has adjusted to her young, overly-playful Boston Terrier sister. Spanky, on the other hand, is thrilled to have Joy.

• One deaf dog owner claims that animals are safer, healthier, and calmer in pairs. Deaf dogs will learn by example from a trained hearing dog.
• Deaf dogs (who live with a hearing, companion dog) "cue off" of the hearing dog–they watch the hearing dog for clues about what is going on around them that they can't hear.

DISCIPLINING

This is a touchy subject, as are most training matters, because some people believe in more physical methods while others believe in more gentle approaches. This is a mix of the two.

• When your puppy is in an off-limits area or object, signal *no* and then give the puppy a "legal" toy or object to play with.
• Tether the puppy to you with a small leash or cord. This way you know where your puppy is at all times and it is less likely to get into trouble.
• Some people believe that correction should be done with a rolled up newspaper, especially with the deaf dog because your hands are for signing and love.
• The following punishments are in order of increasing severity:
    • ignoring - only effective in certain circumstances
    • grabbing the muzzle and glaring pointedly into his eyes
    • a very light cuff under the chin - never hit the nose itself, don't use this often, and be sure to be quick and bring your hand up so it isn't confused with a hand reaching to pet.

• grabbing the folds of skin on the neck and shaking while making hostile eye contact

• alpha roll over - grab neck folds, flip onto back, glare, and hold until he stops struggling and submits. This is a last resort and should only be used when you think your dog is challenging your dominance/authority.

DROP

• Have a treat in the hand that you will use to take the toy. Sign "drop" with the other hand. Your dog will have to drop the toy to take the treat. Give the reward and clap.

GROWLING

Growling is a defensive behavior that signals that a dog feels threatened and anxious. This piece of advice should help.

• Lyndsay Patten, founder of the Deaf Dog Newsletter shared his experience when his dog growled at him: "Cairo growled at me because he was afraid I would take his chew toy away. The solution is to reduce the anxiety and so avoid the defensive behavior (growling). With many dogs, giving a correction will have the opposite effect, reinforcing the anxiety. The approach I used was to approach Cairo not quite to the point where he started to tense, give him a treat, and walk away. With each successive approach I was able to get closer before Cairo started getting tense. After a while I could walk up and pet him and give him a treat without any tension or growling.

"Once you get to the stage where your dog is completely relaxed with your approaching and petting, you can work on actually taking the chew toy away. Try starting with showing the dog that you have a treat, trading the treat for the chew toy, and then giving the chew toy back. After the dog is completely comfortable with you, do the same exercises with other people approaching.

"The important thing is not to push the dog too far too fast, for this to work you have to go at the dog's pace, no matter how slow that is. If you approach to the point where tension or growl results, you've going too fast. With Cairo we overcame the problem in a couple of days, if the behavior/anxiety has become ingrained it may take much longer."

HEELING

Proper leash etiquette is a must for the deaf dog because they spend so much of their life on a leash. Heeling was a simple command for Spanky to learn.

• Sit or stand your dog on your left. Brush your left hand parallel with the left side of his face and move your hand forward in a sweeping motion. As you move your hand, start off with your left foot (the leg beside her). Have a food reward in your hand so she moves forward at once. Reward. Once you are sure she has the signal down, you can reward less frequently. She will eventually learn to start with just the movement of your left leg. Note, when you leave her and expect her to stay, you start off on the opposite leg.
• To "halt," stop walking with a very gentle and slight shake on the leash.

HOUSETRAINING

This is a very lengthy topic and there are many techniques used to teach dogs to do their business outside. With the deaf dog, use an appropriate sign (the ASL sign for "out" is to hold the right hand inside of the left hand and pull it upward and out. Some owners use two hands rolling around each other.) Two to three days of total concentration on housetraining helps the dog to get the message, but housetraining is about a three month process.

Remember, it is the responsibility of the owner to take the dog out, especially in the beginning. Anticipate your dog's needs. Don't wait until you see him squatting to go on the floor. Basic tips follow:

• The very best advice I have to offer anybody training a puppy or dog is to take your pet outside every 20 minutes and stay outside until they go. Develop a hand sign to signal your dog that this is the business they are to attend to. They usually need about 15 minutes to go through the bathroom ritual (finding a place and actually going). When the dog does his business, praise and praise and praise. Food rewards are appropriate in the beginning training stages.
• Choose a particular place outside the house for the dog to use. Always walk the dog to that spot.
• Tie your dog to you on a seven to ten foot leash or cord when you are at home so you can keep a closer eye on your dog.
• If your dog does his business in the house, pick it up with paper and place it outside in the area where you want your dog to use. Calmly show it to your dog.

66

• If the dog squats and starts to go, stomp your foot, gently pick the dog up and take it outside.

• If accidents continue to happen, seek medical advice. There may be a physical problem that is undetectable, such as cystitis.

IDENTIFYING AND INTRODUCING YOUR DOG
Advice on how to prevent your dog from getting lost and how to be prepared if he does.

• Buy a dog tag stating, "_____ is deaf. Please hold and call: your name/ phone number."

• One deaf dog owner ties a scarf on her dog that says, "deaf dog," to inform strangers from afar.

• Visit the folks in your neighborhood. Show them a picture of your dog (or take him with you). Give them a colored index card with your dog's name, your name, your address and phone number. Explain that your dog is deaf and is always on a dog run or fenced, but should he ever get loose, you would appreciate their calling you.

• If your yard is fenced, and there is need for the meter people to get in the yard (my electric meter was in Spanky's fenced backyard), post a sign on the gate: "Attention, please! Our deaf dog is fenced for its own protection against traffic. Please be sure that the gate is securely closed when you enter and leave." I also contacted the utility company and asked if I could send a poster with her picture, our address, and the deaf dog and closed gate information on it. They posted it on the bulletin board so that anyone substituting for our regular meter man would also know. They were very cooperative.

• If your dog is not fenced, always alert any delivery people about your dog's deafness. Ask them to pay special attention to its whereabouts when they move their vehicle.

• A fellow owner highly recommends the tattoo or microchip for identification of your pet. She has a strong point when she says that a tag can be removed.

JUMPING
This behavior can startle strangers. Teaching your dog not to jump on people is a basic step in keeping aggression in check, not to mention, common canine courtesy.

• Have the dog on leash when visitors are coming in or people are approaching your dog. If the dog tries to jump, tell him no. When he settles, praise.
• Always have your dog in a sitting position when guests are entering your house. Teach guest the sign for *get down*.
• When walking and someone is approaching, get out of their direct path and have your dog sit. When the person has passed you, reward quietly and resume your walk.
• Keep a treat box by the door. Reward your dog with a treat when he sits and stays on command. Give a treat to your visitor to give to your dog.
• When your dog jumps up on you , hold on to front feet and walk the dog back like a wheelbarrow. After a few steps, sign "no" and let go of her feet.

LEASH TRAINING

The leash is a way of life for a deaf dog. That's why it is so important that your dog learn to walk on a leash in a manner that is comfortable for both of you. Never walk your dog in a high traffic area without a leash. The deaf dog has no way of hearing oncoming traffic.

• The leash is not a tool for restraining your dog, instead you will find it is a great tool for communicating. When Spanky and I are walking, I gently jiggle the leash to signal her that I am turning around or to give her a sign.
• Pinch Collars only look cruel, according to one member. It is used for correcting the dog when pulling on his leash. The collar, when properly used, improves communication, is nearly impossible to slip out of, and can grow with your dog.
• If your dog pulls, turn and walk in the opposite direction taking the dog with you. When the dog almost reaches the end of the leash going this direction, turn and walk the opposite direction once more. It helps call their attention to you and encourages them to follow rather than try to lead.
• Simply stop walking and freeze until the dog stops pulling. Resume the walk. When the dog pulls again, stop again. Repeat until the dog catches on. This may make for some long (time-wise) walks, but the dog does eventually learn.
• Wrap the leash around the dog's body in this manner: Put your dog on your left, take the leash (and use a buckle collar not a choke) and put it around the body by going to the "outside" under the chest (behind the front legs) and bring it up on the "inside" (between you and him) then to keep it in place, pass the leash under the snap where it is attached to the collar. What happens is when he

pulls, the leash tightens around the rib cage and applies the pressure there instead of on the neck.

• Keep the leash between his front legs which stops any pressure on his throat and makes him very easy to control (pulling on the leash lifts his front leg).

• These collars have been recommended by deaf dog owners as effective against their dogs pulling on their leashes: the Four Paws No Pull Collar, Promise Collar, Halti Collar, Gentle Leader.

LOCATING YOUR DOG

Sometimes trying to find your dog in the house or outside can be maddening. I have found that keeping a bell on Spanky's collar helps me locate her. Keep in mind, however, it doesn't work unless your dog is on the move.

• Put a bell on your dog. Hunting dog bells are good, but if your dog is too small for this size bell, use Christmas bells. They come in several sizes. You can wire one to hang like a tag.

• Make a bell collar for the best noise making. Sew several to a nylon collar so it can be removed whenever the noise becomes bothersome at day's end.

PETTING

Because a deaf dog looks up at your hands for communication, moving an open hand downward on a dogs head to pet him must be confusing. It blocks their vision when they are looking for a sign.

• Pet your dog under the chin. This makes eye contact possible and that's very important for a deaf dog. Advise others to do the same. Hearing dogs also seem to prefer this way of petting. Let the dog first sniff your hand, palm-up and flat.

• Advise people not to pet your dog from behind. Make sure the dog knows he is going to be touched.

REWARDS

I believe that food rewards are a must in the beginning when training a deaf dog or puppy because it helps you get and keep your dog's attention. Later, food rewards can be reduced. Use other methods of praise such as petting, clapping, playing, etc.

• Carrots, begging strips, dog jerky
• Dalmatians have special dietary needs because of their Purine problem. These food rewards meet those special needs and still qualify as treats: Cheese Whiz, peanuts, raisins, and peanut butter to train and on occasion turkey.

SEPARATION ANXIETY

Remember this simple fact. When a deaf dog can't see you, he can't hear you and as a result, it is as if you have vanished. How many of us deaf dog owners shower with the door open or with the dog sleeping on a rug outside the shower? It is even more difficult for them when we leave the house. These tips can help reassure your dog and keep him calm when you go.

• Give your dog a favorite toy or chewy that will occupy him for quite a while. When you return, greet your dog happily and take him out to use the bathroom.
• Exercise your dog before you leave.
• One member of the Deaf Dog Mailing List says a companion dog helped keep her deaf dog calmer about her absences.
• When I am getting ready to leave (changing clothes, putting on makeup), Spanky sits in my room watching me. I can sense she is a bit anxious so I let her know immediately if this is a trip on which she can go, or if she will have to stay home. If she can go, I give her the *car* sign. If she can't, I sign *stay*. I believe this helps her adjust long before I leave when she isn't going with me. If the reverse is true, she enjoys the excitement and anticipation of knowing she is going. She is also lots of fun to watch as she runs around the house telling everyone she get to go with mom.
• When I leave Spanky, I always turn and signal *good girl* and hold one up one finger to signal *I'll be back. Wait.*
Just a note: Because I have begun traveling on a regular basis in the last year, Spanky has learned that when the suitcases come out, Mom is going to be gone a long time (dog time). She has taken to climbing into the suitcase and sleeping, believing, I suppose, that she will get to go with me. Again, I let her know she will have to stay using the *stay* sign.

SIT, LIE DOWN AND STAY
Start your training with *sit* and *lie down*. Spend about 10 to 15 minutes on *sit*.

Sign *sit*, push your dog's rump down to a sitting position, reward with a treat and/or touch. Repeat 5-10 times and your dog should catch on. Advance to *down* in the same session. With your dog in the sitting position, sign *down* (palm flat facing the ground and moving downward in front of your dog). Holding a treat between index finger and thumb helped Spanky to follow my hand's movement and also tended to help her move to the down position. Repeat 5-10 times.

To teach your dog to sit and stay, give the dog the *sit* command. When your dog sits, use the *stay* command and back away two to three steps. Call the dog to you with the *come* sign and reward. Repeat several times. When your dog has the hang of this, do a sit and stay and turn your back and walk several steps away. Turn to face your dog, release with a *come* signal and reward. Repeat 5-10 times.

Work with your dog on these three obedience commands 10 to 15 minutes daily. Choose the same place to work.

SIT AND STAY MANNERS

This command and learned behavior is a must in a well-mannered dog. It is important for the dog's safety (many dogs are taught to sit and stay at curbs when walking with their owners).

• Sit-stay at the door, in all circumstances. This is how I taught Spanky not to bolt out the door when the door was opened.
• When you have given your dog a sit and stay, as you walk away lead off with your right leg. Remember leading off with your left is part of the heel command and would signal for your dog to follow.
• Sit and stay will help curb jumping when a visitor enters your home or you encounter people on a walk.

SMELL AND SIGHT

As in deaf humans, deaf animals compensate for their inability to hear with highly developed senses of smell, sight and feel/touch. When someone enters the house and Spanky is not awakened by the vibrations or the air pressure change from the door opening, she wakes up within minutes because she smells someone is here. She can find food on the counter and sit exactly beneath it although she is too small to see the top of the counter.

Light, dark, movement and reflections are a constant source of stimulus for her. She seems to see everything, and her peripheral vision is amazing. When your pet appears to be imagining things, ask yourself if it smells or sees something you don't. I know once Spanky barked endlessly out the front door. After almost ten minutes of trying to see what she was seeing, I realized it was the leaves blowing on the dogwood in the front yard.

She notices if anything is out of place in a room or if an object has been moved or a new object placed in a room. Until she grows accustomed to a change like this, she will bark and bark at the out-of-place or new object. I once moved a bird bath to a new flower bed I created in the garden, and it took her quite a while to adjust. I often pick her up, hold her close and walk slowly to the changed area and let her check it out from the safety of mom's arms. That usually helps her adjust much more quickly.

Another topic among deaf dog owners is our dog's reaction to darkness. I wouldn't say that Spanky is afraid of the dark, but her world changes dramatically when night falls and her primary sense is deprived. To go outside at night, she prefers that I am with her. (see Vibrations in this chapter)

SOCIALIZATION AND TOUCH

Socialization should begin with the breeder. But if your dog did not come from a reputable breeder or if you didn't get your dog as a puppy, it's never too late.

Research shows that dogs who are exposed to and experience life with humans between three to five weeks are less cautious and more able to cope. A puppy used to the sounds of household appliances, the television, visitors and other pets are better prepared and less likely to bite or display aggression than a puppy who is isolated without exposure to the world and all its distractions.

Socializing your pet helps the dog to become attached to your family, and accepting of other people and animals. To your dog, your family is its pack, and proper socialization will teach the dog that they are a subordinate member of the family. This will keep bad habits and behavior associated with dominance or aggression minimized. Because males have a greater tendency to want to become dominant at maturity, it is especially important that you socialize a male dog. Everyone in the family must participate in socializing your pet. Children should be a part of the process with adult supervision. Make these activities part of your dog's normal, daily routine.

Handling your deaf dog will help reduce startle reactions. Spanky has been held, patted, stroked, rubbed, scratched, hugged and held close since she was tiny. It now seems that her primary purpose in life is to be touched, followed closely by her intense desire to play toss or tug.

• While the puppy is small, pick it up frequently. Make being held a pleasant experience for the dog.
• Look into the dog's eyes until it looks away from you.
• Rub the dog's stomach while it is on its back.
• Massage your dog with mild pressure from head to tail as it rests.
• During play, don't allow your dog to stand on or over you. A paw placed over your wrist when tugging on a toy is a sign of dominance. Do not allow it.
• Avoid excessive tugging games. At a minimum, they are okay, but it is best to encourage and teach your dog to fetch and drop.
• Teach the dog to sit. Then teach the dog to stay. It is important that your dog learns that you give the commands and they follow them.
• Practice taking food away at mealtimes. Practice with the commands: sit and drop. Praise your dog for complying. Do this only briefly. Do not make it a stressful, threatening situation.
• Gently wake your dog from sleep. Have your dog move from its sleeping spot. Praise and reward when it minds you.
• Teach your dog to give up a toy on command.
• Praise and talk (or sign) in a positive way to your dog, even when the dog is resting or sitting quietly.
• As you pet your dog, gently, but firmly manipulate its ears, paws and mouth.
• Give your dog a command before every activity. For example, have your dog sit before you feed, play, go outside.
• Learn effective and appropriate discipline methods. Use them consistently and remember, positive reinforcement of good behavior is vital. Ignoring bad behavior can usually work instead of physical punishment.
• Develop trust, love and respect with your dog.
• Introduce your friends and family members to your dog.
• Take your dog out with you to the park, outdoor markets, to your children's ball games, and walking in the neighborhood.

SOUNDS

Many of us deaf dogs owners have noticed that our dogs are quite vocal. Spanky makes high pitched whines (some sound like "meow," and others like a child crying). Another member has observed moaning and groaning sounds while sleeping or being hugged. Still other have reported their dogs howl, and like Spanky, move their mouths while whining which looks like and sounds like your dog is talking back to you. It's a very funny sight and sound! I have also heard several owners say their dogs are very loud when they eat and drink. Some of this may be breed related, and some not.

STEALING TREATS

Because treating the deaf dog is an important reward system in training the deaf dog, it is important that they respect you as the rewarder and that they not assume the role of snitch.

• Hold one hand under your dog's chin when presenting a treat. If your dog tries to snap the treat away, withhold the treat. The presence of the hand under the chin helps hold the dog's head still to prevent your dog from stealing the treat or reward.

WAKING YOUR DOG

"Let a sleeping dog lie." Sage advice, especially when the dog is deaf. Waking a deaf dog is a common cause of startle response and biting. That's why the following information is vital to your dog's peace of mind and good nature. For a while, give a treat every time you wake him. When the startle response begins to diminish, ask visitors to wake the dog with the method you have chosen to use. To wake your dog, try any of the following. However, when you find the most suitable method, use it consistently and teach your family and friends the method. I highly recommend you insist that children never touch or go close to your dog while it is sleeping.

• Softly blow in the dog's face.
• Touch the dog gently in the same place (shoulder is best).
• Put your hand in front of your dog's nose, or stand close by and let your smell wake her.

74

- Give her a treat every time you wake her. The treat will make waking up less traumatic and she will take eager instead of angry.
- Stomp your foot.
- If it is after daylight, try turning a light off and on. Spanky is less irritable at bedtime when I use this method.
- Gently shake the cushion or bed on which your dog is sleeping.

VETERINARIAN VISITS

Spanky gets really scared when she visits the veterinarian as do many deaf dogs I have heard about. I take along her favorite treats for the vet, techs and assistants to give to her. It is very important that the veterinarian and his staff understand that your dog is deaf and that they are accepting and supportive. Many vets hold to the old way of thinking that all deaf dogs should be euthanized. If your vet believes that way, or in any way makes you feel uncomfortable, change veterinarians. One owner recently reported that the vet and staff at an emergency clinic made fun of her dog when they thought she couldn't hear them. Not only is this rude, it is unprofessional.

- When your dog is a pup, a friendly, preliminary visit to the office will help avoid their first visit being filled with unpleasant activities. Call the office to arrange a convenient time to drop by and let your dog meet the doctor and staff.

VIBRATIONS

Many people (including me) are convinced that their dogs can hear a little bit even after they are known to be deaf. Why? Because as the dogs get older, they get even more sensitive to vibrations and sound waves. If a car pulls into your driveway, or someone walks onto the porch, you might see your dog respond. Sometimes a door opening will wake or alert Spanky to someone entering or leaving. I believe it is the change or draw on the air pressure in the room. I have observed Spanky jump and then bark when someone claps or shouts loudly in the same room she is. In this situation, I believe she is feeling the sound waves. Note too, that when a door opens your dog may be alerted. They are also very keen to pressure changes. Vibrations, sound waves and changes in pressure are all things to which a hearing dog may pay little or no attention.

Again, I remind you: I am not an expert dog trainer or behaviorist. I have simply learned by being a dog owner all of my life, and a deaf dog owner for almost three years. The preceding safety and training tips are from hundreds of other deaf dog owners and myself. I cannot stress enough that if you have specific training problems with your deaf dog, buy a training book, consult a trainer or behaviorist, and/or sign up for a training class. Training the deaf dog is the same as training a hearing dog with the exception of using signs to communicate rather than spoken words.

A WORD ABOUT TRAINING HUMANS:
HOW TO BE A RESPONSIBLE DOG OWNER

To commit to care for a pet is as serious a commitment as caring for a child... and lasts almost as long. There are many attributes to a responsible owner, and listed below, you will find a compilation of points I gathered through experience, research, and from fellow deaf dog owners.

• As the owner of a deaf dog, you must have a willingness to learn ASL or other signs to communicate with your dog, and seek a better understanding of deafness in general. You must also have the extra patience and understanding that a deaf dog needs.
• Understand that a dog is for life (a 10-16 year commitment). They are not a disposable item. They are living, feeling creatures who depend on you for training, guidance, love and companionship.
• One must be committed in their responsibilities. (Taking care of pets should be on the same level as taking care of children.)
• Give your dog plenty of love, attention and understanding (just like a child).
• Return the love your dog gives to you. Remember your dog is part of your

pack and you are the leader of the pack. He respects and loves you and wants your approval and acceptance.

• Have a properly secured area for your dog, and always walk the dog on a leash.

• When walking your dog, always clean up after your dog.

• When your dog is on leash, lead your dog around potentially dangerous situations (i.e., other dogs not on leash, traffic)

• Proper identification on the pet (tags, microchip in neck/shoulder area or tattoo: inside hind leg.) Be sure your tag tells of your dog's deafness.

• Choose a caring, concerned veterinarian and be sure they are accepting and understanding of deafness in dogs (or are willing to learn).

• Stay current with vaccinations, flea and heartworm protection, and tend to your dog's health care needs.

• Feed and water your dog. Your dog needs fresh water at least twice each day.

• Properly socialize your dog for your dog's peace of mind, personality and coping skills. This will also broaden your dog's world of friends.

• Properly train your dog. This will make your dog more lovable, sociable, and desirable to be with. Responsible owners train their dogs for manners and manageability. Seek out a "treat and reward" type of dog trainer and avoid any punishment-types of training.

• Educate yourself by reading, researching and talking to other dog owners.

• Spay and neuter your dog at the earliest, safe date (usually 6 months).

• Be patient with your dog. They have bad days, sometimes don't understand what you want, and are occasionally just plain mischievous.

• Give your dog the opportunity to play and interact with other dogs.

• Outside dogs need shade in the summer and plenty of water.

• Brush your dog's teeth to cut down on disease and bad breath

• Never leave a dog alone overnight. If you do go out for the evening, leave lights on for your dog.

The number of pups registered with the American Kennel Club in 1996 alone was 1,332,557! Because there are so many puppies born each year, they have become a disposable commodity if they don't live up to certain standards.

CHAPTER SIX

The Right To Live–
Life and the Pursuit of Happiness

Apply the Dal deaf statistics (12%) to the beloved *101 Dalmatians*.
Of these happy, playful puppies, 12 would be deaf in both ears and would be
euthanized. While this famous litter is fictional, the example demonstrates a
harsh reality. And many of those who can't follow through with the destruction
of the animal often abandon them at a pound or on a country road.

WHY ARE DEAF DOGS DESTROYED?

The culling and destruction of dogs with undesirable traits is common
practice. To justify the practice of culling deaf dogs, the reputation of aggression has become attached to the deaf dog. But with the prior discussions in
Chapter Two, we must ask ourselves if aggression in deaf dogs is fact or myth.

The breeders also insist it is to prevent the continuation of the "deaf
gene" however, spaying and neutering is a simpler and more humane way of
dealing with that problem. And besides, if breeders wanted to end or (at the
very least) curb congenital deafness, certainly they would learn and practice
sound and responsible genetic breeding practices.

As I see it, the biggest problem is overpopulation. The number of pups
registered with the American Kennel Club in 1996 alone was 1,332,557!
Because so many puppies are born each year, they have become a disposable

commodity if they don't live up to certain standards. After all, there are plenty to choose from.

HOW MANY DEAF DOGS ARE DESTROYED EACH YEAR?

While no printed number exists, calculations can be made for the Dalmatian breed based on the number of Dal pups born each year.

In the April issue of *Dog World*, Elaine Waldorf Gewirtz wrote an article on Dalmatians in which she stated "about 12%" of Dal pups are deaf. The latest AKC Gazette litter registration statistics reflects 11,012 litters of Dal pups registered in 1996, ranking the breed 18th overall. If you assume an average of 11 pups per litter (Dals have litters of 8-15 pups), that means approximately 121,132 Dalmatian pups were born in 1996 alone!

The Dalmatian Club of America Board of Governors feels "very strongly that deaf pups should never be sold, placed or given away, and most certainly should not be bred...with the enormous surplus of unwanted dogs in this country, there is no need to preserve dogs with problems such as deafness." If all Dalmatian breeders followed this stance of the Board of Governors of the Dalmatian Club of America, approximately 14,500 deaf Dalmatian pups were born and disposed of in 1996 alone. Culled. Put to sleep. Euthanized. Destroyed. And keep in mind, that is only one breed out of 64 with reported congenital deafness!

Beverly Cuddy, Editor and Publisher of Britain's *Dogs Today* magazine stated, "If you're not a responsible enough breeder to find homes for your deaf puppies, you should not be breeding. Why breed when you know you are going to kill a certain percentage of your litter? I don't understand how these people sleep at night."

WHAT IS THE SOLUTION?

Certainly improving the knowledge of breeders on the subject of genetics and what causes deafness would help tremendously. But unfortunately, not all breeders approach their business with the same ethics and love for animals. The so-called "puppymill breeders" do not approach the breeding business with the ethics reflected by many of the world's top breeders. They are motivated by love of money, not the love of a breed.

Dr. Strain reports these findings that could positively affect the number of deaf puppies born by breeders. "When the piebald gene is strongly expressed it suppresses pigment cells (melanocytes), so you get blue eyes (iris pigment suppressed) and deafness, because pigment cells are necessary for the survival of the blood vessels in the cochlea. Statistically, blue eyed dogs are more likely to be deaf than brown. When the piebald gene is weakly expressed, it does not completely cover up the underlying color (black or liver) and a patch results. Statistically, dogs with a patch are less likely to be deaf. I have reported this in my past publications. The blue eye is not allowed in the breed standard for Europe (or Canada), which may explain why the incidence of deafness is lower there. When breeders breed away from patches, their numbers of deaf dogs increase. The patch is not allowed in the breed standard." So if Dalmatian breeders REALLY want to reduce deafness in their breed, shouldn't the standard disallow blue eyes and permit patches? Note: The desirable pups are born solid white and develop their spots over time. A patch is a Dal pup *born* with a spot that grows into a large patch rather than a spot. In my opinion, the patched Dals are beautiful dogs. In the breed standard, however, they are unacceptable.

The following solution has also been submitted to the AKC and the DCA that could partially solve the problem of deafness in Dals: have all registered Dalmatians tested via BAER, and only permit bilaterally-hearing dogs to be registered. That would prevent unilaterally-deaf dogs (who often sire more bilaterally-deaf pups) from being registered and bred.

Lynn Sickenger recommended another good suggestion. She believes that the growing population of deaf dogs would be better controlled if purebred deaf canines were neutered and registered with the AKC. That would enable the AKC to spot breeders who produce successive generations of deaf offspring and take the necessary steps to stop them from further contaminating the gene pool. Lynn made her point when she concluded, "As it is now, the killing of purebred deaf pups is no different than burning the evidence of a crime."

Lyndsay Patten of the Deaf Dog Web page posted recently, "There is a movement afoot within the Dalmatian Club of America (DCA) to revisit the deaf Dal position; witness the Great Phoenix Dalmatian Club's Deafness Survey in the February issue of the *Spotter*, the DCA's official newsletter." My research has shown that not all DCA members agree with the clubs credo to destroy deaf dogs, but they dare not let themselves be known.

Hearing registries allow breeders to voluntarily have their dog BAER tested. Dogs who have no hearing impairment qualify for certification. The same type of registries exist for hip dysplasia and eye diseases. Hearing registries have been established by the English Setter and Jack Russell clubs, and at long last, the Dalmatian Club of America is in the process of putting a hearing registry in place.

The hearing registry won't solve the problem, nor will the deafness survey being done by the Great Phoenix Dalmatian Club, but it is a step in the right direction.

CAN DEAF DOGS COMPETE IN OBEDIENCE TRIALS?

Having never been an enthusiast for dog competitions, this is unfamiliar territory for me. I have, however, done some research and inquiries and have come up with several organizations who do allow deaf dogs in their competitions. For those owners who wish to get their dogs involved in competitions, these groups will welcome their participation.

On the North American Continent, deaf dogs are allowed into the following obedience trial and agility competitions:

• United Kennel Club (UKC)
100 East Kilgore Road/Kalamazoo, MI 49001
Website: http://www.ptialaska.net/~pkalbaug/ukcindex.html

• American Mixed Breed Obedience Registry (AMBOR)
AMBOR Competition Program/Mr. Tim Elkins
8616 Lochdale/Dearborn Heights, MI 48127
Website: http://member.aol.com/amborlcr/ambor/home.htm
E-Mail: AMBOR Main Office @aol.com

• Canadian Kennel Club (CKC)
Commerce Park, 89 Skyway Ave/Suite 100/Etobicoke, Ontario
Canada/M9W6R4/Phone (416) 675-5511/FAX (416) 675-6506

• North American Dog Agility Council, Inc. (NADAC)
HCR2 Box 277/St. Maries, ID 83861
http://www.teleport.com/~jhagland/nadachom.htm.

• United States Dog Agility Association
P.O. Box 850955/Richardson, TX 75085
Phone (972) 231-2700/FAX (972) 503-0161
E-mail: info@usdaa.com   Website: http://www.usdaa.com

NOTE: Many of the same types of organizations exist throughout Europe and
Australia that allow deaf dogs to compete.

While some clubs welcome the deaf dog into their competitions, the
largest kennel club in the United States, the American Kennel Club, does not.

In *Dog World* magazine, author Mary Thurston told of a 7 year old
Dalmatian (now retired) who competed in AKC competitions all over the
country. She placed consistently among the top dogs. But had anyone discovered that the dog was deaf, her obedience ring days would have been over.

The AKC Statement of Purpose reads, "The basic objective of Obedience Trials is to produce dogs that have been trained and conditioned always to
behave in the home, in public places, and in the presence of other dogs, in a
manner that will reflect credit on the sport of obedience." Their general regula-
tions bar blind or deaf dogs from competing "in any Obedience Trial or Tracking Test or Tracking Dog Excellent Test, and must be disqualified."

There have been few to challenge their stance, but Lynn Sickenger,
owner of a deaf Dalmatian known as Dickens, took them on single-handedly in
the early 1990's. Her basic logic was that, "People would be furious if the
Olympics barred deaf athletes from competitions. Deaf dogs should have the
same right to compete against their hearing peers."

In her letter to the AKC in the Fall of 1992, Lynn stated that obedience
trials are based solely on performance "No special concessions would need to
be made by the judge, and the handler would use hand signals which currently
are acceptable to the AKC. Although deaf dogs may not hear distractions in the
ring, their other senses are more acute. For example, my dog sees everything,
from small insects to flashes of light that you or I would never notice. A deaf
dog's enhanced sensitivity to outside visual stimuli more than offsets any
benefits from not having sound distractions in the ring." Lynn's letter resulted
in the AKC advisory committee voting unanimously to recommend to the AKC
board of directors that the rule barring deaf dogs from the obedience ring be

changed. The Dalmatian Club of America recommended that the AKC board disregard the recommendations of the advisory committee. Certainly this, and perhaps other influences were factors they considered when they voted against the deaf dog's right to compete in AKC obedience trials in the fall of 1993.

If you are the owner of a deaf dog and wish to address this issue with the AKC, send your letters to: American Kennel Club/Board of Directors/51 Madison Avenue/New York City, New York 10010.

WHAT OTHER CERTIFICATIONS AND OPPORTUNITIES ARE AVAILABLE FOR THE DEAF DOG?

Many of the members of the Deaf Dog Mailing List have Canine Good Citizen certificates for their dogs. This is a noncompetitive, onetime evaluation of the dog's behavior in public, around strangers and other dogs, and around distractions. For an information pack, write to:

• Canine Good Citizen Certificates (CGC)
American Kennel Club/CGC Program
5580 Centerview Drive #200/Raleigh, NC 27606

Some deaf dog owners have involved their dogs as volunteers visiting the sick and elderly. For information, contact:

• Therapy Dog, Inc.
P.O. Box 2786/Cheyenne, Wyoming 82003
Phone (307) 638-3223
Website: http://home.ptd.net/~compndog/tdi.html

CHAPTER SEVEN

In Their Own Words

Deaf Dog Owners
Introduce Their Dogs
And Share Their Stories

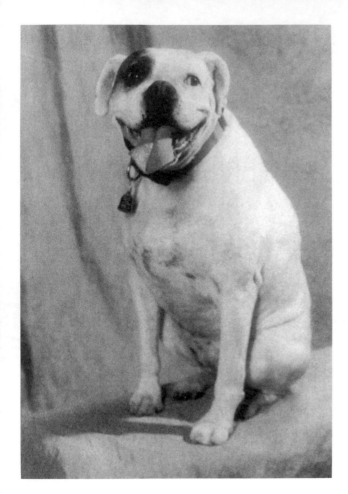

HEIDI

Breed: Boxer
Owners: Julie and
Doug Nelson
Tennessee

Heidi adopted us. Doug found her wandering around at the airport with a large black dog when she was just a few months old. He brought her home and we fell in love with her.

We did not realize she was deaf until we'd had her for a few weeks. She started out sleeping in the garage and we would pull the car into the garage (it's a loud diesel engine), slam the car door, and then walk right by her bed and she wouldn't move a muscle. We both thought she was really a sound sleeper. It didn't occur to us until later that she might be deaf.

We then took her to a local veterinarian for shots and asked him to check her for deafness. We expected she would be hooked up to complicated monitors to test her hearing, but when we picked her up that day, the vet said, "Oh, yes, we stood in back of her and

clapped our hands and she didn't turn around so, yes, she's deaf."
We did not know about the BAER test and our vet did not refer us,
so this test was never done on Heidi.

Because we are so crazy about this dog, there was never any
question about keeping her or not. She became part of our family
from the first day. Deafness just didn't matter.

To train Heidi, we used signs we invented. For instance, we wave
our hands to get her attention and then point where we want her to
go or sit or whatever. She always knows what we mean and what
we want. At night we have had some success with flashing the
porch light to get her attention. We are careful never to let Heidi
out when not on a leash or in a fenced area.

We don't believe Heidi is handicapped at all by her deafness. She's
very smart and seems to have enhanced senses that more than
make up for her deafness. Never give up on a dog just because it
can't hear you. Deaf dogs are wonderful pets and can teach a
family a lot about life. We wouldn't trade Heidi for the most
pedigreed hearing dog anywhere. She is a unique and wonderful
dog.

When Heidi was about 18 months old, she brought Red, a golden
retriever, home with her one day. She seemed to be telling us that
Red was going to be living with us from now on and sure enough,
he's still here. Heidi watches him and barks when he barks, chases
birds when he does...we believe Red is Heidi's "hearing-ear dog."
He is very patient with Heidi and seems content to help her with
things she can't hear for herself. Her barking does seem to get on
his nerves sometimes. Since she can't hear herself bark, she barks
VERY loudly, never gives up and will stand and bark at the back
door for as long as it takes to be let in.

SEURAT

Breed: Dalmatian
Owners: Gina and Greg Brockway
Pennsylvania

I was working as a veterinary technician when a breeder brought
this puppy in to be euthanized because it was deaf. The vet in

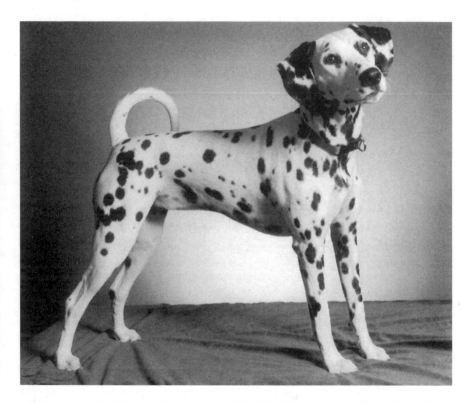

charge asked the breeder to give the puppy to me. When I took her
and held her in my arms, she began to wriggle and licked my face
all over. She gazed lovingly into my eyes and then snuggled into
my neck. I couldn't let this puppy, so full of love and life, be
senselessly destroyed.

90

To train Seurat, I looked in the library for information on training a deaf dog and talked with an obedience trainer–all to no avail. Finally, I did it all on my own. When I discovered the Internet, I exchanged advice and ideas with a few people. We used carrots as rewards, used hand signals to communicate, a lot of touching for praise, and a squirt bottle for reprimands. To call her, we stomp our foot on the floor twice. She learned quickly to turn and look for the source and she now relates it with us calling her.

The biggest handicap to the owner of a deaf dog how to call the dog to you from long distances. But the biggest benefit is the close bond between owner and dog because of the increased attention and touching that is needed in praising the dog.

The most important training tip I can offer is don't ever give up! Be patient. Be creative. Teach your dog to accept being startled without reacting (as deaf dogs have a tendency to do). From the time Seurat was a puppy, we purposefully startled her awake and then lavished petting on her if she didn't snap. This taught her not to lash out in fear when she becomes startled. Don't think of deafness as a handicap. It's a gateway to another realm of companionship. You need to be more aware of and responsive to your dog, and your dog will do the same. I don't believe in striking any dog, but especially not a deaf dog. Your hands are one of the most important tools of communication between you and your dog.

Seurat is VERY sensitive to smells. I might be able to sneak to bed past the other sleeping dogs but not Seurat. While the hearing dogs continue to sleep, Seurat leaps up and stands at the top of the stairs as I head to bed. After many different attempts, we've decided it must be our scent wafting to her that wakens her. We can wake her up simply by holding a hand in front of her nose...no movement, no touch...just our scent. And skunks drive her bonkers!

BAILEY

Breed: Great Dane
Owners: Sandy Suarez Boutin and Jim Boutin
Michigan

We knew Bailey was deaf when we adopted her from a Great Dane
Rescue. Jim and I felt that Great Dane Rescue would have a hard
time finding a good home for Bailey, so once we saw her she was
ours. She is truly a beautiful, loving, intelligent companion.

Since we couldn't find a book on training deaf dogs, and knowing
Dalmatians have a high incidence of deafness, we called the
Dalmatian Club of America for advice. They were amazed we
had adopted a deaf dog. They recommended we put her to sleep as
soon as possible and told us she would go crazy when she got
older! We have since called them back to tell them what a wonderful pet she is, but alas, they don't return our calls.

To train her, we invented our own signs, observed the signs she
responded to and used those signs faithfully. We signed, showed
her what to do, and rewarded her. She sits, lays, comes, and has
even taught herself how to open the door and let herself outside.
To get her attention, we tap her on the shoulder or point to her.

The only real danger I can think of that the deaf dog and owner
face is if they are off leash. As a result, Bailey is NEVER off
leash. As a safety precaution, she wears a bell on her collar in case
she were to get away from us or out of the fence, we would hear
her bell.

The most important training advice we can offer is to be patient.
The dog might be deaf, but certainly is not stupid. Stick to one
sign for one command.

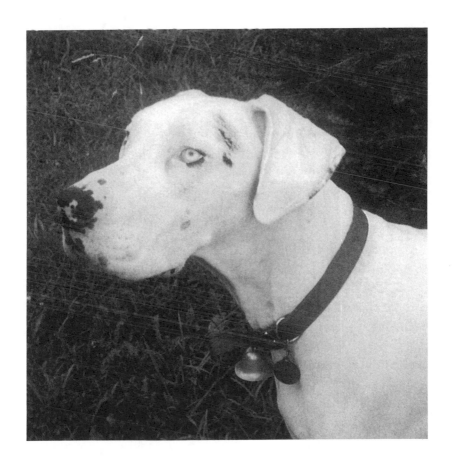

Don't listen to breed clubs, breeders or vets if they tell you to put your dog to sleep. Listen to your heart. All Dane and Dalmatian breeders "put down" their deaf puppies because they feel handicapped dogs are a "misrepresentation" of the breed.

We have three Danes. Ashley, who is "normal," Bailey who is deaf, and Beau who is blind (by an accident). It is so cute the way they play together. Beau can always find Bailey because of her bell ringing. Bailey has no idea how he finds her since she can't hear her bell. Bailey also tries to sneak up on Ashley (with her bell ringing all the while) and gets a confused look on her face when Ashley turns to look at her.

SPOT

Breed: English Cocker Spaniel
Owners: Wendy Royston
Ontario, Canada

Spot's breeder was aware he and a sister were deaf and looked for homes willing to give them the love and extra attention they would need. The decision to take Spot was a tough one. Our yard is not fenced, and the trainers I contacted for advice were not helpful. But we agreed to meet the puppy and it was love at first sight.

The first place I turned to for training instruction was a local highly respected obedience school. After an expensive private lesson, they said Spot could never work in a regular obedience class because he was deaf and would be too disruptive to the class. The second kennel I dealt with had the same attitude, but I finally found help at the local kennel club's obedience classes. The trainers there said we would learn together, and after 16 weeks of training, Spot was ready to move on to agility training. We use standard obedience signs and ones we make up, most of which come naturally. While we have never signed his name, a "Queen Elizabeth" wave will bring him running.

The biggest handicap we experienced was finding a trainer. Most were less than willing to expand their limits, experience and education to include the deaf dog. This surprised me since I had assisted in an obedience class where we had two deaf sheepdogs. These two had the highest marks of all the dogs in the class because they had to pay close attention to receive their commands.

Benefits? The bonding that takes place between the deaf dog and its owner is stronger because of the eye contact. As a groomer by trade, I take Spot to malls to demonstrate my craft, and to hotels for overnight seminars and competitions. During these outings, he is so relaxed. Nothing fazes him. The people at the mall can call him as much as they like, but he doesn't hear and, therefore, ignores them. He falls asleep on the grooming table and rides up and down on crowded elevators, taking everything in stride.

When we were working on recall in training class, the instructor took Spot, turned their back to me and began feeding him weiners (and as you know, a dog would sell his mother for food). I went to the other side of the room, jumped up and down and waved my arms (my sign for "come, Spot") and he came immediately leaving the weiners behind. I don't know who was more surprised...me or the trainer!

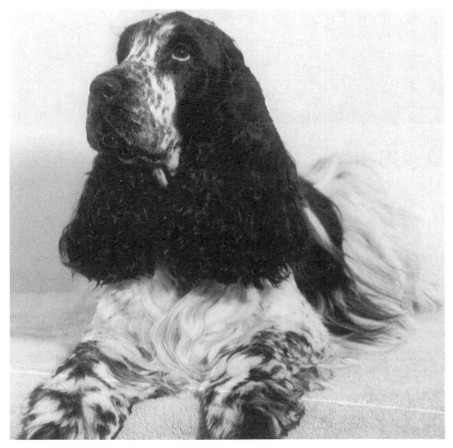

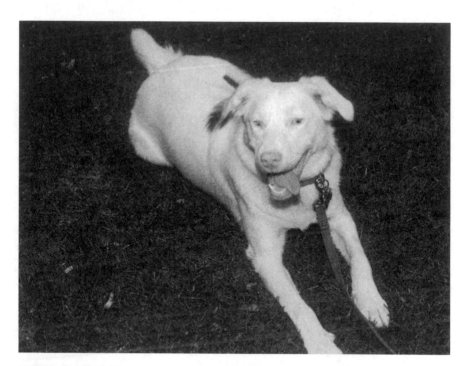

WOOF

Breed: Mixed
Owner: Marcy Rauch
White Plains, NY

Woof is ten years old and what I lovingly call an Abomination Shepherd (part albino Australian Shepherd). I adopted her from the SPCA, and while I knew she was deaf, she was the cutest, most responsive puppy there. All I had to do was make eye contact with her for her to respond.

To begin her training, I took her to puppy kindergarten. I was lucky enough to get a trainer that worked with high level obedience training and had also trained a few deaf dogs. Woof ate the diploma on the way home.

Woof learned standard obedience signals and signs that I invented. I don't sign her name, but stomp the floor or flick the lights on and off to get her attention. I have heard of some deaf dog owners who use flashlights, but for some reason, Woof is terrified of flashlights.

Being owned by a deaf dog is a mixed blessing. Having been an animal lover and owner my whole life, I have to say that I have never had a bond quite like this one. Woof and I need each other in a special way.

I recommend to anyone who owns a deaf dog that they love and communicate with them as best they can. Obedience training is very important. And talk to your dog. Woof can read my expressions as well as my body language. I've been talking to her, laughing at/with her for the past ten years. Being deaf only means the dog can't hear. Not that the dog can't understand.

Last summer, Woof became very ill. She was paralyzed from the neck down (cause was never fully determined), but I was told she may never walk again, and if she did, it would take months. They didn't know the resolve of a dog who had to spend her life pushing the limits to understand the rest of the world. Within a week, she took her first step. And now, one year later, she rollerblades with me, staying in heel position and senses where everybody and everything is around her with that extrasensory "whatever" she has that compensates for her deafness.

On a lighter note, I have an old beat up station wagon for hauling the dogs, groceries, etc. The car is known as the Woof Wagon. Woof sticks her nose out the window and sings with the vibrations of the bass lines of the radio. It's embarrassing sometimes, since the sounds coming out of my car are so loud and off key that people turn around to see who's beating up a dog.

SPOTTY

Breed: Dalmatian
Owner: Carol Barwick
Gordon, Tasmania, Australia

I have four children and my youngest child was born deaf. She is 17 and uses sign language to communicate. We have become part of the deaf community and have met some lovely people. Two years ago, we had a phone call from the Tasmanian Deaf Society asking us if we would be interested in a deaf Dalmatian. We had just lost our German Shepherd, but still had our Pekinese and cat.

My daughter Leearna kept asking us to have a look at this pup. She was so worried that it would be put to sleep if no one gave it a home.

We got the name and number of the breeders and went off to meet the next night. When Leearna picked up little Spotty, there was a special bond straight away between them because they had something special together– they were both deaf. So after all our instructions on food, health care and agreeing to have Spotty

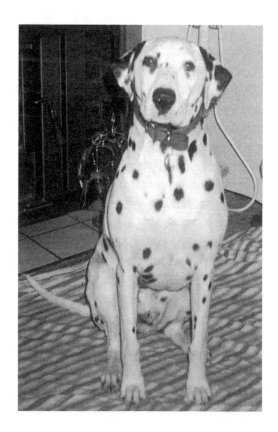

desexed, we went home with Leearna and Spotty cuddled together.

We started to sign to Spotty straight away so that he would know to watch our hands. We showed him around his new home and introduced him to the other animals who not very impressed with this bundle of energy that wanted to play with them.

It didn't take long to toilet train him and for him to learn what the sign was for "toilet." He got to know where he was allowed to go and where he wasn't. He loves to run over to the horses and play. He also knows he is only allowed to go down the driveway when he is with someone. He enjoys a walk to the jetty and loves the beach.

As he grew he learned more signs. He is two years old now and has grown into a lovely strong dog. He loves people and likes to be around us and have lots of cuddles. We have had to be firm with him so he knows discipline. He has been very easy to train and has not shown any violence to anyone or any of our animals. (His only fault: when he is walking on a lead, he is very unfriendly to other dogs. Otherwise, he loves to play with other dogs at our home or the beach.)

Spotty loves balls and loves to play chasing in a circle. He has three different barks: one when he has lost his ball and wants someone to get it; another is when he can't see you (he barks until he spots you; and the other is his big brave bark when he stands on the veranda and thinks he is king.

I find it very hard to accept that anyone can put a deaf pup to sleep. We don't do that to deaf children. No one can completely stop deaf puppies from being born, but we can learn to love and accept them and not put them down. They have a right to live life to the fullest. All they need is patience, time and love.

KELLIE

Breed: Border Collie
Owner: Lesley Bustard
Northallerton, North Yorkshire, England

Kellie was born into a litter of four puppies I bred that were sired
by Obedience Champion Lymewell Skipper. Two days before she
was to go to her new home, I was doing some housework and
noticed that while the other three puppies had shot into the pen she
laid still, fast asleep. I realized she must be deaf. When my vet X-
rayed her, he found damage to two cervical vertebrae consistent
with her having run headlong into something. She was then
hearing tested which confirmed that she was bilaterally deaf. The
vet who tested her advised me to have her put to sleep. I had
already made up my mind that was not an option.

Having had dogs all of my life and competed in Obedience for 16
years, I have a lot of experience in training dogs. I sat down with
my friend and worked out the commands I would need for everything I wanted to teach her from basic household obedience to
competition work. I decided from the outset I would compete with
her if she took to it, and enjoyed that side of training.

I think what helped me most is that I am handicapped myself. I
have a lateral curve of the spine. I tried to give to Kellie all the
things my Mother gave to me in terms of freedom and a spirit to
overcome difficulties.

From the first, Kellie enjoyed her training. I made no allowances
for her deafness. She was praised when she was good and told off
when she was bad! We coined a phrase for when she had just not
understood what I was asking her to do–she's deaf, not daft! She
always tries so hard to please me. When things went wrong and I
knew it was me and not her, I would sit down on the floor and

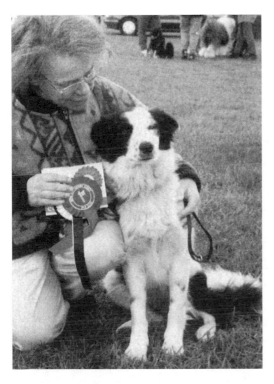

cuddle her, tell her by my breathing and hands that it was OK and not her fault. Then we'd try again. I spent a lot of time playing with her and teaching her everything that a hearing puppy would learn. She went everywhere with me because I felt it was very important for her to see and understand that the big wide world was nothing to be afraid of.

Some people in the Obedience world thought I was mad to try competing with her, but she took so well to training. It took me less than five minutes to teach her the sign for "sit." Because she depends so much on her eyes, our training sessions had to be short. I talk to her, because saying the words helps my face give off the right signal too.

Our relationship is wonderful. She is always near me and I'm sure it is not just because she is deaf. She gets on well with my other two dogs.

1995 was our first season of competition and we finished it with 5 second places in Novice Class, 2 fourths, 2 fifths and a sixth place. This season she has had 3 first places, 1 second, 1 third, 2 fourths, 2 sixths, a seventh and a ninth from 15 competitions. I am over the moon with her. Several people in the know have said she has the ability to go all the way.

INCA

Breed: Boxer
Owner: Christine Wingate-Wynne
Totton, Southampton, England

Inca's breeders were considering having her put to sleep, but I never thought twice about adopting her. I am partially deaf myself and whilst appreciating that dogs and humans are different, my parents did not say they did not want me because I was deaf. We brought her home when she was nine weeks old. We already had Mitzi, a crossbreed, who was not happy about the situation initially, but after two years, accepts Inca as a buddy. I promised

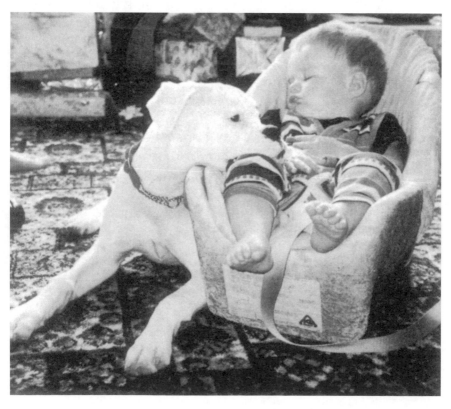

myself if Inca showed any distress or depression due to her deafness, I would have to face facts and consider having her put to sleep. I was, however, going to give Inca a chance of a good life, and hopefully prove the skeptics wrong. Because I have learned in my life that deafness or a hearing loss can cause isolation, I felt Mitzi was important to have around for Inca. She gives Inca clues as to what is happening–people approaching or that Marc's home, or a cat's come into the garden.

Marc and I attend the Solent and District Dog Training Club with Mitzi and began taking Inca right away. As Inca and I have progressed with training, I have worked out a series of hand signals which Inca responds to best. In December, 1993 at the Dog's Club annual bash, Inca won the Best Progress award at nine months old. At two and a half, Inca reached grade five at the club which is the top class. And in December,1995, she won the club's "Tara Cup for Agility Superstar."

When we introduced Inca to walking on lead, we used a lead that was half chain, half leather. The chain is nearest her mouth, so that chewing the lead never became a problem. With regards to hand signals, these were made up as we progressed with training. Using friendly reward training and making sure the dog follows your hand is invaluable.

Inca greatly enjoys going to the Dog Club and she is not satisfied until she has said hello to all her admirers. The admirers, in return for saying hello to her, receive some very big licks and cuddles. She is an extremely social dog. She has a great love of life and enjoys meeting people whether adults or children. The photo of Inca is an example. When my napping nephew was put on the floor in his seat, Inca placed her ball on his lap and waited patiently for him to throw it. I believe Inca is a great example of why we should not write off deaf dogs.

FRANKIE

Breed: Dalmatian
Owner: Mr. Holmes and Mr. Burba
Brighton, East Sussex, England

Frankie was born into a litter of pups we bred. When we saw her beautiful blue eyes, we could do nothing but keep her. We welcomed the challenge of raising a deaf dog. She has a fantastic nature with everyone every other animal she has ever met. And we think she's the most beautiful dog you'll ever see.

We spoke to Lyn Diable at Kushti in West Sussex for training advice. We trained her ourselves, which was a bit of a challenge, and we had our ups and downs. We tried different ideas until we eventually found the way that worked best for us.

We used hand signals, but mainly experimented with facial expressions, and always treated when training. She also learned a lot from our other two Dalmatians. We used signs we invented to get her attention or call her: we wiggle our fingers at her and she comes to us. She is such an affectionate and loving dog an owner could ever wish for.

We have found the following to be very important in training and communicating with a deaf dog: 1) build up trust with your dog; 2) get the dog used to being around other dogs, crowds and traffic; 3) be strict in training your dog, but also loving because the dog has more trust in you than you know or realize; 4) enjoy your dog...even if deaf, the dog has all the usual needs of a hearing dog.

One day, when Frankie was younger, we had all been for a walk and Cherrie (Frankie's mom) began to limp. When we arrived home and inspected, she had a cut on one of her pads. We cleaned it up and put some cream and a dressing on it. All the time,

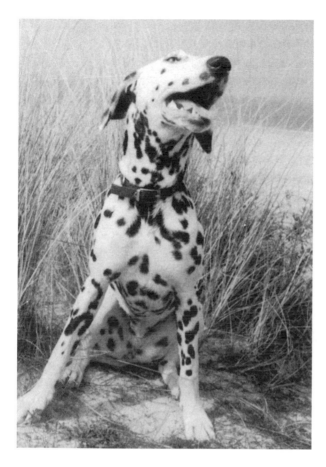

Frankie was sitting and watching very patiently. The moment I finished, she moved up to me with her paw held up. I shook it, as if to say hello, but this did not please our little Frankie. She wanted some cream and a bandage too! And of course, she got her way.

She loves to sleep with the cats, and she can often be seen sleeping with one of two of them curled up around her face. She seems to like this as she always sleeps with her head either buried under something, often her own legs as if she prefers sleeping so the light does not disturb her.

So many people are under the impression that it is cruel to keep a deaf dog alive, let alone have one in a family as a pet. Nothing could be further from the truth. Our experience and life with Frankie is that the love, affection and devotion from a deaf dog is rare and special.

Afterword

Deaf dogs face lots of uncertainty when they come into this world. Some don't leave the veterinary clinic after the BAER test is administered. There are those who are abandoned or dropped off at the pound. Some of these orphans are rescued and loved. Others are not. But those who are given a chance at life with patient, conscientious owners, live life as beloved, family pets.

Living with a deaf dog has enriched the lives of many people all over the world. The special bond between pet and master is enriched by the incredible trust and communication that develops.

When I asked deaf dog owners about this on my research questionnaire, I received responses that were universally felt.

- "I believe the dog's deafness brings owner and dog closer, because you bond with a handicapped dog in a way you might not with a hearing dog. They are more dependent on you."
- "We have a wonderful relationship. It's difficult to explain but she is always near me."
- "I think we've developed more patience, and we're a little more understanding of deafness in general."
- "There is a closeness and a bond between owner and pet."
- "Deaf dogs are wonderful pets and can teach a family much about loving and living."
- "Owning a deaf dog has helped me become comfortable communicating with deaf people. It has opened up a whole new world for me."

As owners of deaf dogs, we seem to agree that living with a deaf dog constantly teaches us the importance of communication, trust, tolerance, love and patience.

In short, living with a deaf dog constantly teaches us how to be a little more human.

...this research can remove the myths of aggression and brain damage, and move the deaf dog forward in acceptance in the canine world.

Research/A Request for Input and Information

This book is the first of its kind. And that's why I am using it as a forum to request information from deaf dog owners, trainers, veterinarians, behaviorists, breeders and other dog lovers for their experiences and knowledge.

My request for input and information will help to continue and expand research on deaf dogs: their lives, habits, training, personalities and temperaments. This data will be used to compile facts, figures and statistics that give a clear and honest look at deaf dogs. I will share my data with Dr. George Strain of LSU and any other professional or organization in the field who is interested and/or working in the field of canine deafness. I do this because I believe the deaf dog is a noble, trustworthy animal who deserves a chance at life; and that this research can help remove the myths of aggression and brain damage, and move the deaf dog forward in acceptance in the canine world.

ON THE TOPIC OF TEMPERAMENT AND AGGRESSION

Up until very recently, when deaf dogs have been written about "aggression" is the buzz word. But in all of my research, I could document but ten cases of aggression involving a deaf dog. One of my goals is to compile all of the information about aggression incidences so that a solid set of statistics can be calculated based on written accounts that have been collected and compiled. I believe that only then will deaf dogs get a fair chance.

If you are interested in participating in the collection of information on Deaf Canine Temperament, please complete Section B of the questionnaire. Both non-aggressive and aggressive behavior reports are invited. If you have already filled out a questionnaire, complete the questions that were not on the original survey and it will be attached to the one I have on file from you.

Thanks in advance to all of you for any information or stories you provide. This is the method I used to gather the knowledge and experiences that have been shared in *Living With a Deaf Dog*. Hopefully, this book and input from you will be the foundation that will help open the hearts and minds of others to these wonderful animals.

Mail questionnaires and correspondence to: Susan Cope Becker/Deaf Dog Research/2555 Newtown Road/Cincinnati, OH 45244
E-mail address: scope2000@aol.com

DEAF DOG OWNER QUESTIONNAIRE

SECTION ONE/BASIC INFORMATION AND INPUT

1. Your Name, Address (regular mail and E-mail), Phone, FAX
2. Pet's Name, Breed, Birth Year, Sex
3. Did you buy or adopt your pet and how long have you had him/her?
4. Did you know your dog was deaf when you got him/her? If yes, why did you decide to adopt/buy/keep a deaf animal? If no, when and how did you discover your pet was deaf?
5. Do you own other pets. Describe. (please include any handicaps)
6. Did you have the BAER (brainstem auditory evoked response) test performed on your dog? If yes, where?
7. Where did you turn for advice on how to train your dog?
8. Are you usually a dog/pet owner? How did you train your dog? Do you have experience training a hearing dog?
9. What are the five most important training tips you would like to share?
10. To train did you use: a.) American Sign Language b.) Standard Obedience Signals c.) Signs you invented
11. How do you sign your dog's name or signal for him/her?
12. What negatives do you find with your dog's deafness?
13. In your opinion, what positives are associated with your dog's deafness?
14. Please share a story or particular experience you have had with your dog.
15. Please finish with any additional comments, stories, tops or experiences you would like to share.
16. Would you agree for your self and your dog to be photographed, quoted and/or written about in future deaf dog books written by Susan Cope Becker? If so, please state at the end of your questionnaire and sign.
17. Are you a breeder, trainer, veterinarian, veterinary student, deaf dog owner?

SECTION TWO/TEMPERAMENT, TRAITS AND PERSONALITY

1. Has your dog shown signs of aggression? i.e., biting, growling, attacking
2. If so, please complete the following:
   a. Was the dog eating, sleeping, startled?
   b. Who did it involve? (i.e. children, strangers, other dogs, family)

c. How old was your dog when this happened?

d. Where did it happen?

e. Was anyone hurt?

f. How did you manage and discipline the dog?

h. Did you keep your dog?

i. What measures did/do you take to prevent a reoccurrence?

3. Have you or anyone you know ever been bitten or attacked by a deaf dog? If so, please describe the incident, relating all the details asked for in question 2.

4. Does your dog ever growl at you or others? Please explain.

5. Specifically, how does your dog behave around children?

6. If, in your opinion, deaf dogs are not aggressive, please share your reasons and experiences. Share also how you believe dominance in a dog can be overcome especially if you have experience with this.

SECTION THREE

SPECIAL AWARDS OR ACCOMPLISHMENTS

1. Is your dog certified by Good Canine Citizen or as a therapy dog? Please share some experiences your dog has in their work.

2. Does your dog compete in agility or obedience trials? With what organization? What awards has your dog won?

3. Has your dog been recognized in the media as a deaf dog for an outstanding achievement or heroics?

4. Is your dog a celebrity? Has he/she been featured on television or other media (local or national) for their work or abilities?

5. Does your dog have a web site? Please share the address.

• FEEL FREE TO ADD ANY SUGGESTIONS, COMMENTS OR INFORMATION YOU FEEL IS IMPORTANT.

• IF YOU HAVE A PHOTO OF YOU AND YOUR DOG OR OF YOUR DOG, PLEASE SEND IT ALONG WITH YOUR QUESTIONNAIRE (PHOTOS CANNOT BE RETURNED).

• COPIES OF ARTICLES, NAME AND DATES OF TV SHOWS GREATLY APPRECIATED. (VIDEOS OF TV IF YOU CAN SPARE A COPY)

RESOURCES

DEAF DOGS MAILING LIST

The Deaf Dogs mailing list is intended to be a resource for people who live with deaf dogs, and those otherwise interested in deaf dogs. The list is not moderated, the only taboo topic is advocating that deaf dogs be euthanized.

To subscribe, send an introduction to deafdogs-request@cybervision.com. It can be as short or as long as you like. The suggested minimum content is to give your name, your dog's name, how long you and your dog have been together, and what topics you are interested in discussing. When asking questions on the newsletter, be sure to be specific.

THE DEAF DOG WEB PAGE

On this web site you will find a list of training tips and written hand signs to use when training and communicating with the deaf dog, personal stories from deaf dog owners, and other deaf dog related information and links.
http://www.kwic.net/~cairo/deaf.html

DEAF DOGS WITH THEIR OWN WEB PAGES

• Cairo's Page   http://www.cybervision.com/~cairo/
• Lady's Page   http://www2.eastlink.net/user/djricke/dals.htm
• Maggie-Mae's Page   http://www.htcomp.net/zap/maggin.index.htm
• Jack Russell   http://www.cis.ohio-state.edu/~wreid/wishbone/
• Sweetpea on the White Boxer Page   http://boxerworld.com/whiteboxer/
• Cricket   http://www.geocities.com/heartland/plains/9576/index.html
• Chief Kelly   http://www.neca.com/~bhdavis/linda/linda.html
• Pongo and Hallie   http://www.geocities.com/heartland/hills/1819
• MacAbee Pet   http://www.mailexcite.com

DEAFNESS IN DOGS AND CATS WEBSITE

Dr. George Strain's (of Louisiana State University) web page. Provides thorough genetics discussions on canine deafness. Many links to other deaf dog sites.
http://www.lsu.edu/guests/senate/public_html/deaf.htm

DEAF DOG ORGANIZATIONS
• Deaf Dog Education Action Fund
PO BOX 369, Boonville, CA 95415

E-mail: DDEAF @aol.com

Founded in July of 1997, the Deaf Dog Education Action Fund's goals are to provide new deaf dog owner with free training information. They are a non-profit organization that will also work to educate the public about canine deafness and the nature of deaf dogs to help create a better understanding and acceptance of these animals. They also have a listing of deaf dogs who need homes and potential owners who are seeking a deaf dog to adopt. DDEAF also assists in finding donated transport for such animals. Donations welcome. T-shirts and bumper stickers for sale. Opportunities for membership and volunteer positions are available. For more information, contact Holly Newstead at DDEAF@aol.com. Visit their web site at www.deafdogs.org

• Kushti Dalmatian Club and Animal Sanctuary
Lyn Diable/Nutshell Farm/Cophatch Road/Rusper/West Sussex RH 124RR/ England/Phone 01293 871247 FAX 01293 871123

Lyn and Paul Diable breed Dalmatians, as well as shelter, train and place orphaned Dals, hearing and deaf. With such a large undertaking, they are always looking for contributions of old blankets for bedding. This group takes a strong stand in ending euthanasia of deaf dogs by Britain's Dalmatian club. Donations help feed, train, relocate and save deaf Dals.

• Santa Fe School for Deaf Dalmatians
P.O. Box 8921/Santa Fe, New Mexico 87504

Caroline Crosby has trained and placed deaf Dalmatians since 1992. Write for their booklet, Deaf Dalmatians: Ownership and Training. Donations help feed, train, relocate and save deaf Dals.

PRODUCTS RECOMMENDED BY DEAF DOG OWNERS
Harnesses and Leads
• Halti Leads

• No-jump Harness (one owner referred us to 1-800-JEFFERS for this product)

• Lupi Harness

- Gentle Leader Head Halters
- Tri-Tronics Collar

Inquire about vibrating collar. May only have a low shock collar.
- Barking Collars that emit citronella when the dog barks.

RECOMMENDED READING BY DEAF DOG OWNERS
- Tufts University monthly newsletter, *YOUR DOG.* Subscribe for $30 a year by writing to Your Dog, PO Box 420272, Palm Coast, FL 32142-0272, or call 1-800-829-5116.
- Clicker Training books and videos by Karen Pryor or Gary Wilkes
- *Hear! Hear! A Guide to Training a Deaf Puppy* by Barry Eaton
- *Good Owners Great Dogs* by Kilcommons & Wilson
- *How To Raise a Puppy You Can Live With* by Rutherford & Neil
- *The Dog Who Loved Too Much* by Dr. Nicholas Dodman
- *Caesar: On Deaf Ears* by Loren Spiotta-DiMare (a charming children's book)

* These canine magazines also recommended: *Dog World, Dogs Today, Off-Lead Dog Training.* Available in most bookstores.

DOG RESCUE WEB ADDRESSES
http://www.freenet.msp.mn.us/people/shaffes/rescue.html
http://www.pstbbs.com/tammyb/dog/
http://www.pioneernet/sucia/
http://www.akc.org/rescue.htm
http://www.ddc.com/rescue/dane

MAGAZINE ARTICLES
DogWorld, Magazine/April, 1998 Editorial by Editor, Donna Marcel
Dog Fancy Magazine/May, 1998 Breaking the Silence by Don Vaughan
Pets Magazine/March, April, 1998 Caring For a Deaf Dog, by N. Glenn Perrett

NOTE: These books, magazines and products have been found useful by deaf dog owners in training and communicating with their deaf dog. This list does not reflect any endorsement by the author of these products (addresses or sources are listed only if available at the time this list was created.)

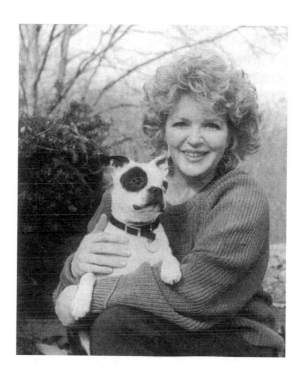

Designer, writer and dreamer, Susan Cope Becker is the creator of Pibbles, a thought-for-the-day cartoon, and numerous advertising campaigns, television commercials and videos. She is an avid journal keeper and has taught journaling classes since 1983.

Susan was chosen by Yoko Ono to edit and design two greeting card lines: John Lennon's greeting cards, *Imagine*, and Yoko's cards, *Dream Series*.

She makes her home in Cincinnati, Ohio with her husband, Ethan Becker, the author of the new *Joy Of Cooking*. They enjoy gardening, hiking and reading. They often escape to their cabin the mountains of East Tennessee where they share time in the kitchen, in the woods, and on the porch.

Ethan and Susan have two grown sons, David Cope and John Becker. They share their home with Spanky, a congenitally deaf Boston Terrier, and Joy, a selectively deaf German Short-Hair Pointer.